£20.

	DATE DUE	
JAN 3 1 1991		
OCT 1 3 1992		
DEC 1 4 1993		
APR 0 4 1997		
OCT 2 3 2003		

MANAGEMENT AND ADMINISTRATION
OF REHABILITATION PROGRAMMES

REHABILITATION EDUCATION: A SERIES IN
DEVELOPMENTAL HANDICAP

Edited by Roy I. Brown, University of Calgary

*VOLUME 1: INTEGRATED PROGRAMMES FOR
HANDICAPPED ADOLESCENTS AND ADULTS*
Edited by Roy I. Brown
(Croom Helm, London; Nichols Publishing Company,
New York, 1984)

*VOLUME 2 : MANAGEMENT AND ADMINISTRATION
OF REHABILITATION PROGRAMMES*
Edited by Roy I. Brown
(Croom Helm, London; College-Hill Press, San Diego, 1986)

Management and Administration of Rehabilitation Programmes

Edited by Roy I. Brown

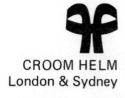

CROOM HELM
London & Sydney

©1986 Roy I. Brown
Croom Helm Ltd, Provident House, Burrell Row,
Beckenham, Kent BR3 1AT
Croom Helm Australia Pty Ltd, Suite 4, 6th Floor,
64-76 Kippax Street, Surry Hills, NSW 2010, Australia

British Library Cataloguing in Publication Data

Management and administration of rehabilitation
    programmes. – (Rehabilitation
    education)
    1. Rehabilitation
    I. Brown, Roy. II. Series
    362.4'048   RM930
    ISBN 0-7099-3916-7

Printed and bound in Great Britain by Mackays of Chatham Ltd, Kent

CONTENTS

PREFACE

ACKNOWLEDGEMENT

Roy I. Brown, Professor and Head, Department
of Educational Psychology, and Coordinator,
Rehabilitation Studies, The University of
Calgary, Calgary, Alberta, Canada

Peter R. Johnson, Davies & Johnson Associates,
Psychoeducational Services, Delta, British
Columbia, Canada

Keith F. Kennett, Dean, School of Education,
Nepean College of Advanced Education, Kingswood,
New South Wales, Australia

Roy I. Brown, Professor and Head, Department
of Educational Psychology, and Coordinator,
Rehabilitation Studies, The University of
Calgary, Calgary, Alberta, Canada

Peter R. Johnson, Davies & Johnson Associates,
Psychoeducational Services, Delta, British
Columbia, Canada

This book is the second in a series in the field of Rehabilitation Education. It is argued that in behavioural, social, education and allied areas, principles of rehabilitation are similar throughout a wide range of disabilities. Services, policies and programmes must reflect the needs of people with disabilities. But policies, management and programmes frequently diverge from these goals. Thus administration and management must be redirected towards the individual concerns of disabled persons, and to do this it is critical to examine rehabilitation philosophy and the means by which such philosophy is put into action.

The book begins with a series of chapters directed to the improvement and refinment of management and service delivery within rehabilitation agencies. Some practical guidance is provided on ways in which such development can take place. Rehabilitation Education is providing a platform through which new and innovative approaches can be considered. Several chapters are directed to this end. The reader will find some differences in approach and philosophy, but the aim is not to present a totally cohesive picture throughout, but to look at various innovations which may have relevance to the future development of services. This may be done through setting up demonstration and pilot schemes which require careful monitoring and evaluation. The issues of evaluation are discussed.

Finally, there is some discussion regarding staff stress and efficiency, for it is believed that the effectiveness of programmes is partly determined by the psychological health of the staff involved.

The material is directed towards a wide range of professionals, particularly those in psychology, social welfare and education, but also other colleagues in various aspects of the helping professions. In a number of countries students are enrolled in professional programmes for rehabilitation educators, counsellors and practitioners. Some universities and colleges are beginning to create programmes for new professionals. This particular series represents an attempt to deal with some of the issues these practitioners will face as they attempt to develop a new range of programmes for the latter part of this century.

It is hoped that government workers, board members of agencies, and members of advisory committees will consider the arguments and examples seriously, for shared responsibility between consumer or client, and professional worker is a serious proposition. Indeed it is recognized that behavioural change does not represent recovery from a disease, where intervention may sometimes appear separate from personal involvement, but a recognition that behavioural change and development is brought about through the individual's conscious awareness, self concept and motivation. The individual fully participates in the change process. A partnership is required between clients and professionals representing a transdisciplinary organization. There should also be partnership between an agency's board and its staff, as well as conjoint approaches by government and service delivery operations. The theme of this book is therefore partnership within one or more models of service.

R.I.B.

ACKNOWLEDGEMENT

I wish to thank a number of people for helping to prepare this book. The patience of the various authors in dealing with suggestions and concerns in a timely manner is appreciated. They have made a number of revisions which have hopefully created a central thrust to the book.

I am grateful to Mary Brown for her comments on a number of issues in specific chapters, and, in particular, I wish to acknowledge Sister Maureen O'Connell from Australia who, while attending the Rehabilitation Studies Programme, The University of Calgary, read the draft manuscripts and provided many perceptive comments.

Linda Culshaw, who applied herself once again to the task of committing our writing to word processor, has enabled us to produce this volume on time. However, my thanks to her go much further than this, for she ensured letters and agreements, comments and suggestions were faithfully recorded and dealt with in an orderly fashion. Finally, I am grateful to Tim Hardwick of Croom Helm, whose advice and encouragement continues to help make editing this series a pleasant task.

R.I.B.

Chapter One

MANAGEMENT AND ADMINISTRATION IN REHABILITATION: AN
INTRODUCTION

Roy I. Brown and Peter R. Johnson

INTRODUCTION

As indicated in the first volume of this series, rehabilitation education refers to the broad range of programmes
which, from behavioural, educational, and social points of
view, enable children and adults to function increasingly
effectively within society.   Such programmes attempt to
apply   the   philosophy   of   social   role   valorization
(Wolfensberger, 1983).   Social   role   valorization   is   a
development and advance on the often misunderstood and
abused Principle of Normalization. Social role valorization
refers to the esteem associated with many of the roles in
our society. Thus when people with special needs adopt a
positively valued persona, such as that of a skilled worker,
musician, or parent, they benefit from the role's image
enhancing properties.
     The authors believe that the basic principles and rules
put forward in this chapter apply *to all programmes dealing
with people of various ages who have many different types of
handicap*. But our interests are wider than this, for we
also believe the principles, if not the levels of application, apply in different countries despite the fact that
philosophy and management style may differ. The terms that
we use in this chapter are intended to be generic.   The
chapter is concerned with management and administration. It
should be recognized that, although precisely the same board
and management organization or structure may not exist in
each agency, because of different terms of governance, the
concepts discussed apply generally.   If the component
structures are not present in any form, then the agency,
and, therefore, the consumers and the staff are likely to
encounter particular difficulties.
     In Canada the field of rehabilitation is dominated by a
range of agencies which are designated for the most part, as

1

private structures with their own philosophies and independent boards of management. They receive their funding from government, but have charitable status and receive donations and support from a number of other sources. In Britain the agencies are often government structures, relating to local health and social authorities and receiving their funding directly from these bodies. They frequently do not have boards responsible for their direction and running. Yet within the structure of the local authorities are systems which relate to authority and responsibility.

This book discusses a variety of issues concerned with the interface between management and programme development in a range of rehabilitation services. The particular agencies may be associated with government departments or boards of education, health and social services. Some are private foundations or charitable associations. Some may have components which deal with research and hopefully others are recognized as demonstration centres. However, most of them are concerned with the delivery of day-to-day services for people living with one handicap or another.

Education services may be viewed by some as rather different since, in several countries, education of children is required by law, or community school boards generally assume education should be supplied to all children regardless of handicap. We suggest that the majority of recommendations within this book apply equally to educational authorities, private centres, and agencies dealing with children, adolescents and adults. Indeed one of our concerns is that the bureaucratic classification system separating people by age and condition is an administrative convenience which restricts the delivery of effective service to disabled persons, and profoundly influences our ability to apply demonstration and research knowledge to general practice.

It is suggested that the various managements, boards and allied structures, developed within the field of rehabilitation over the past decades, have not adjusted to the knowledge now existing in the behavioural, social and educational sciences and that we have therefore reached a crisis in relation to the management of agencies working in the rehabilitation field. If we are to unravel this problem and come up with helpful recommendations, then it is first necessary to discuss the role of boards, management, and equivalent bodies responsible for overall philosophy.

One problem commonly experienced is that board members or advisory personnel lack an understanding of the role of committees in general and, more specifically, the aims and responsibilities that they may be taking on in relation to the rehabilitation field. Board members should obtain a general knowledge of agency functioning and direction and develop a philosophy in relation to their agency, and their intentions for clients they are serving.

For example Brown and Hughson (1980) have pointed out that problems arise at both conceptual and practical levels in terms of the function of sheltered workshops and vocational training agencies. In theory the programmes for each should be entirely different because the philosophy of the two types of agencies are entirely different, but most members of boards do not recognize this, nor do the agency staff. Unless functions are clarified, problems occur at the frontline level, at board level and, frequently, at the funding level; the latter often represented by government departments. Furthermore, personnel hired to work in a sheltered workshop, activity centre or training agency should differ markedly.

Such a situation occurs in Canada where many government agencies provide funds for day programmes. The funding for the most part ignores whether training or shelter workshop functions are carried on. As a result many individuals or their parents expect to receive a particular type of service, but do not do so because resources are not available. This is very different from saying that resources do not exist, either in terms of knowledge or funding.

Over the past 50 years there has been a considerable growth of knowledge in the rehabilitation field. It is generally recognized (Clarke, 1979) that if we applied our knowledge within our agencies, the amount and degree of handicap, particularly mental handicap, would be much decreased by the end of the century. We recognize that this will not happen, but submit that one of the crucial limitations relates to the structure and management of agencies. We have not yet developed mechanisms for incorporating successful change from demonstration programmes to general agency function. Nor do we have proven structures to move research knowledge to formal agency practice, although in subsequent chapters some possible examples are given. The incorporation of such structures involves changes in staff knowledge and flexibility, the job expectations by and of staff, a clear management philosophy which is client centred and a board which is directly concerned with agency direction.

We will attempt to look at some of the administrative and management qualities which make for the success or failure of a particular agency or centre. In doing so it is necessary to outline some major agency functions.

PHILOSOPHY AND GOALS

Most agencies and organizations have a constitution and a philosophy. Yet, when we have looked at the range of

3

agencies in a variety of countries we find staff are frequently not aware of them and in some cases a written philosophy and constitution does not formally exist! The constitution is a means of describing an agency's purpose and reflects a basic philosophy. It is the basic description of its aim from which all of its activities must be derived. Variations in philosophies and goals can have profound effects on the types of service offered. For example, an agency might be designated as a non-profit making organization whose resources of funding are directed to the care and treatment of individuals with handicaps. Sometimes the principal goals may be quite broad, at other times they are narrow and relate to only one specific type of condition or disability. For example, an agency may be concerned with care or treatment, home living or vocational training, cerebral palsied or mentally handicapped persons, adult accident victims or childhood disabilities, or to a combination of these and other attributes.

An agency might have a goal to rehabilitate handicapped individuals. On the other hand it might have a goal which is directed towards the care and protection of such individuals. It may be much broader and involve integrated programmes covering residencies, home care, leisure time and social education as well as vocational training.

Coordinated programming with a view to integrating people into the community represents a philosophy of social role valorization, and indicates the areas in which environments are to be normalized. But obviously this philosophy can only be effective if it is put into practice by agency personnel.

Although we agree that both agency personnel and boards of directors should be involved in the development of philosophy, the prime responsibility for saying what an agency is about must reside within the latter. Obviously philosophy is not a static function and we recommend that it is looked at continuously. A full appraisal is desirable every one to two years, with a view to ensuring the philosophy is consistent with the most modern knowledge available for rehabilitation purposes. This means a coherent policy, based on discussion involving all facets of staff and board personnel and often involving outside advisory consultants, rather than arbitrary action by the board, manager or executive director.

Many boards do not know the purpose of their agency and, furthermore, staff frequently disagree with one another on the major aims and how the agency should function.

We have reached a time where it is unacceptable for board and staff to belong to an agency on the one hand but have different views and aims at a macro level from the stated philosophy and goals of the centre. For example, it is of little help if personnel in a residential unit do not believe in a normalization philosophy when an individual from this unit is attending a day programme which does believe in integration. Handicapped people are often placed in difficult positions when different approaches are applied to them at different times of the day. This is hard for non-disabled human beings; it is quite intolerable when it is applied to those who have restricted abilities in one field or another.

Prospective staff should be given the constitution and goals to read on application. Disparity or disharmony between these and their own views should be explored and, if crucial, the applicant should be rejected. This is an important aspect of interviewing procedures.

The staff, including the executive director and manager, are responsible for the day-to-day running of the operation. That is their major role. They are also responsible, particularly the senior staff, for the design of programmes and for seeing that the philosophy pervades the programme at a practical level. The arguments above suggest different roles for board and staff, but in many countries the managerial staff are also separated clearly from mid management and frontline staff. There is a clear-cut hierarchical model imposed, with levels of function and responsibility clearly defined. We argue that this is not effective in the running of rehabilitation agencies (see Chapter Five). There is a continuum of activity which involves all levels of staff and board, and although there may be a preponderance of certain types of activity among certain members at particular levels of the continuum, the vast majority of members share functions to a lesser or greater degree. If this line of argument is accepted, it must follow that the board and senior management must be knowledgeable about staff, and agency aims, and the effects the agency is having at a practical level. Without such knowledge they cannot support the effective operation of the agency. Likewise, it is only when the staff understands the philosophy and its programme implications that the delivery of service to specific individuals is likely to be effective.

If a philosophy is to be a dynamic and changing structure, staff and board alike must consciously ensure that it is effectively evaluated on a group basis and changes are made after ratification by senior management and board. Agency reviews are often done by outside personnel. We do not totally concur with this view, although the process may be helpful. It alone can be quite damaging, particularly if the outside consultants are not knowledgeable about the field. This may seem an odd statement, but our experience suggests consultants are not always selected by boards or government departments on a knowledge basis. Other social and political pressures hold sway.

5

It is also important for staff to evaluate their own programmes so that they can become aware of deficiencies and be provided with the authority and direction to eradicate problems. Without this responsibility, agency personnel often blame other authorities for inadequacies and inaccuracies. They also argue that change cannot occur because of rigid bureaucratic authority. Many agencies are stagnant or deteriorate because the agency structure is not such that senior personnel can second authority or permit directional and controlled change to take place. Some of the reasons for this are discussed later.

Simple diagrams, which outline the procedures involved in committee structures, are often helpful to all those involved and give a visual impression not only of philosophy but of line authority and committee requirements. Other aids that can be employed are the recording of interviews with clients about programme and programme needs and the impact that the programme has had on the individual. An example of this was recorded by Brown (1985). Such input is not just important in terms of agency structure but also adds to programme effectiveness. If, for example, one of the aims is social role valorization, it makes sense for clients to be encouraged to make recommendations.

The Voluntary Society

In many countries, it was the parents of handicapped children who established the first community agencies. Many did not wish to send their children to large institutions, but found that local educational services were not available to them. Consequently, groups of parents organized themselves to provide basic schooling for their offspring. Some approached local ministers regarding the use of church basements, while others complained to their elected representatives about the lack of services. While these parents knowingly became the first service providers in many communities, they had perhaps unwittingly embarked upon their most powerful role as advocates for people who live with a handicapping condition (Sarason & Doris, 1979). To this day, service delivery and advocacy remain the dual roles of these voluntary societies.

Over the last 30 years in Australasia, the British Isles, and North America, parent-directed associations, sometimes named for a specific disability, have grown enormously in number and political power, and have provided a range of sophisticated programmes. In some countries, such as Canada, the relationship between societies is that of a *grass roots* movement. Power resides in local groups rather than in any national body. In each geographical area, these locals combine to elect and direct members of a regional body. The regional associations in turn sponsor a national society for handicapped people.

Advisory Boards

It is recognized that many agencies will not have boards as such, or that these boards are remote within some government authority and have very little direct contact with agencies. We advise that such agencies form their own advisory committees which make recommendations directly to local or other government authorities, that they are formally constituted and represent a knowledge base. The following chapter relates to these advisory committees as well as governing boards.

A board of directors is responsible to the general membership for the functioning of the agency and may be responsible to government for the application of funds. It is a means of developing a specific framework for promoting the philosophy and programme base of an agency. Individual board members should recognize that they are on the board for the better functioning of the agency, not to represent personal concerns. Parents sometimes have this conflict and need to recognize their different roles, one as parents of students in the agency and the other as impartial board members. The selection of members to advisory committees is critical. The staffing of an agency and how it develops a board has been described by Brown & Hughson (1980), also Nemeth, Brown and Hughson (1981). However, whether it is a new board or new members are being added to the board, the executive director or manager should ensure that each member has a clear knowledge of the agency and should be able to recognize the common problems and assets which exist. Each member should be provided with a constitution, bylaws and goal statement as well as a brochure describing the functions of the agency. Such documents have other uses for the public as a whole. In addition, short training courses for board directors are most useful. These are available in many cities in North America. A slide presentation of an agency's activity may be of assistance. Board members should be encouraged to visit the agency on a regular basis. However, individual board members only have rights in terms of the agency's constitution and, out of courtesy, should always discuss their visits in advance with the executive director or manager.

In some agencies the executive director or manager is a voting member of the board or advisory committee, on the grounds that they have a major say in the function of the agency and should be regarded as of equal standing in the board structure. Others argue that their influence would be too great, and on this basis, some advisory committees argue that the committee is there to advise the executive director. In order to overcome the voting difficulties, some groups agree to work on the basis of consensus. These different methods are acceptable, having various advantages and disadvantages. It is up to the members to select the method which best suits the agency they represent and to ensure that the responsibilities and functions are clearly written down so that all may know which procedures are acceptable.

It is often useful at such board and senior staff meetings to have more than the executive director or manager present. Another senior representative from staff is often desirable. The argument for this is *the hour-glass effect*. In many agencies the director or manager becomes the only means by which board and staff communication takes place. This is not necessarily an adverse process in the hands of an effective individual but, unless he or she is capable of representing differing views impartially, problems often arise in terms of communication and interpretation. The availability of a second member of the team not only provides for a broader knowledge base, but can be very supportive to the manager or executive director. It also provides a depth to perception which is necessary for all parties concerned.

In broad terms, the board is responsible for the development of philosophy, and the executive is to see that philosophy is carried out. A management committee, chaired by the manager or executive director and made up of senior staff, is responsible for the day-to-day running of the agency and bringing forward recommendations to other committees.

In dealing with the greater community only the executive director and chairperson should be making public statements, otherwise great confusion can result in the public mind and opportunities exist for playing off one subgroup against another. Staff or board members as individuals do not speak for the society, but, on the other hand, staff members must know that they can take issues directly to a member of the senior management group and that there are systems and rights for appeal if events require this.

OVERVIEW TO SUBSEQUENT CHAPTERS

The above outlines some of the issues that confront societies, agencies and their boards, management and personnel. Because they dramatically affect the nature of the organization, they have a major influence on programming opportunities as well as the lives and future of the clients involved. In the subsequent chapters, authors examine different issues arising around the management, administration and programming field. An attempt has been made to compare and contrast various models and to consider some of the advantages and disadvantages of the various organizations. For example, programmes in Israel and United States are examined and compared. The differences that are seen in these programmes may be a feature of *the stage of development* or they may underline particular strengths and weaknesses of the particular programmes. Again, the issues which surround manpower shortages relate clearly to the bureaucratic nature of some programme organizations. Thus it is of interest in some recent work by Brown, Bayer and MacFarlane (1985) that only about one third of the time of frontline supervisors was found to involve individual training or group treatment. Further, the issue of vocational rehabilitation compared with integrated programming for clients comes to the fore. These issues are critical for, whether integrated programming takes place in one agency or in different agencies, they give rise to major philosophical, programme and management issues. It is our concern that many handicapped people are *pulled apart* by the many different forces which act on them. Very often those forces are brought into being by bureaucratic and regulatory procedures, which have more to do with an orderly convenience rather than the needs of specific clients.

An attempt has been made to provide some examination of the major aspects of board and agency structure. Many of the comments made are not put forward as inviolate principles, but guidelines which may be reflected in different ways in different agencies and in different countries. However, without some recognition in each agency of these requirements it is likely that great difficulties will emerge. In the development of agencies, now frequently under pressure of funding contingencies and continual need for client support and assistance, it is recognized that evaluation of programme content and its relationship to management activity must be pursued diligently. Some examples of this are given in the various chapters.

One outcome of rehabilitation is stress and burnout for staff. Such issues are discussed and it is suggested that they, like many other programme features, need to be recognized within the organization and are the concern of knowledgeable managers and board members.

An attempt has been made to introduce some innovative and creative methods of dealing with programme development, yet we suggest that new concepts and ideas must still recognize the need for structure and stability; two factors which are essential if programmes are to result in effective rehabilitation.

We are aware that in a changing age of rehabilitation there are cycles of activity which do not necessarily

reflect a continuous move to integration. Reinstitutional-
ization and sheltered workshop programming may once again
come to the fore and reduce the progressive action that many
countries have experienced over the past few years. The
responsibility for such regression does not lie just with
economic change and political initiative. It is the collective responsibility of well informed board and staff members
who, along with the advocates of people with disabilities,
whether parents or volunteers, to help determine the nature
of advance and change in rehabilitation services.

REFERENCES

Brown, R. I. (1985) 'Programs and Problems in the Field of
    Adult Rehabilitation,' in C. K. Leong & D. C. Duane
    (eds.), *Understanding Learning Disabilities:
    International and Multidisciplinary Views,* Plenum
    Press, New York.
Brown, R. I., Bayer, M. B. & MacFarlane, C. (1985) *Rehab-
    ilitation Programmes Study,* National Welfare Grants
    Program, Health and Welfare Canada.
Brown, R. I. & Hughson, E. A. (1980) *Training of the
    Developmentally Handicapped Adult,* C. C. Thomas,
    Springfield, Illinois.
Clarke, A. D. B. (1979) 'Presidential Address, From
    Research to Practice,' in P. Mittler & J. M. deJong
    (eds.), *Research to Practice in Mental Retardation,*
    University Park Press, Baltimore.
Nemeth, S. L., Brown, R. I. & Hughson, E. A. (1981) *Rural
    Programs Manual,* Special Programs and Resources for
    Kids Society, Calgary, Canada.
Sarason, S. B. & Doris, J. (1979) *Educational Handicap,
    Public Policy and Social History*, Free Press, New York.
Wolfensberger, W. (1983) 'Social Role Valorization: A
    Proposed New Term for the Principle of Normalization,'
    Mental Retardation, 21(6), 234-239.

Chapter Two

MANAGEMENT AND ADMINISTRATION IN REHABILITATION: ROLE OF
VOLUNTARY AGENCIES AND THEIR BOARDS

Keith F. Kennett

INTRODUCTION

The management and administration of programmes are
essential components in the effective delivery of
rehabilitation services. They can be divided into two major
categories:

1)   the overall policy-making, and
2)   general strategies and the daily routine of
      implementation.

A board of management, sometimes called a voluntary agency
board, is the senior body responsible for decision-making,
policy and action that gives direction and opportunity for
agency development.
      The purpose and final responsibility for the quality of
services rests with the board of directors, who must
delineate programme priorities and provide clear statements
of objectives, agreed upon by both themselves and the
employees. Specific goals and strategies are essential for
the sound delivery of professional services, and the success
of efficient fund-raising projects.
      The final responsibility and the power of decision-
making and direction for the development and service
afforded by the agency rests with an elected group of people
- board members or directors - whose major qualifications
for such responsibility are generally their willingness to
stand for office, and a membership willing to elect them.
      Voluntary agency boards are essential and how they act
is critical. The possible effectiveness of such action is
examined in relation to the calibre of the directors and
their abilities to control and initiate events. Various
committees are discussed, a model is presented for a person-
committee fit, an examination is made of the importance of

11

motivation and quality management, and suggestions are given for effectiveness of communication among all components of the organization.

An agency needs a collective purpose, which involves a partnership between directors (board members) and professionals and can only be accomplished by effective communication. Increased efficiency in programme delivery and rewarding professional experiences rely upon ease of communication amongst the board, senior employees and the total team of professional and administrative staff. Thus, an understanding of the specific roles and responsibilities of individual directors and the board as a whole are necessary in any dialogue on the management and administration of rehabilitation services. Nowadays, such responsibilities demand adaptive behaviour by board members, who may need to take risks in order to seek new solutions to old problems.

BOARD AND DIRECTORS

Purposeful and Vital Directors

Purposeful and vital directors attempt to ensure the success of a voluntary agency board when, by encouragement and co-operation, and strong support, they allow professional, administrative and fundraising staff to focus their attention and energies on the essential services. Under the competent leadership of a president, supported by informed and supportive board members, the voluntary agency board sets the tone, the harmony, and the vitality that assures purpose and participation in attaining pre-determined goals and ongoing services.

A competent voluntary agency board gives a sense of well-being, a meaningful and well-explained philosophy, security to employees, financial viability, and a pre-determined structure of events within the overall framework of forward planning. Such action is taken to provide a firm foundation upon which a voluntary agency meets the prime purpose of its existence, namely to maintain and improve professional services.

Prime Purpose: To Maintain and Improve Professional Services

The prime purpose of all those involved in a voluntary agency is to maintain necessary programmes and improve professional services. The realization of this aim depends on the degree to which board directors, administrators, fund-raisers, members, involved families, friends and the professionals consider their efforts as a joint venture. Professional staff must focus on monitoring, evaluating and improving programmes, especially in terms of individual development, personal and social attainments and adaptive behaviour.

The voluntary agency board is of prime importance in the success, enjoyment and satisfaction of both service suppliers (agency personnel) and service receivers (clients). The success depends not merely on discussion, monthly meetings and signing cheques, but on consistent and purposeful action and effective results. Conversely, inaction is the quickest way for a voluntary board to collapse through inertia and disorganization.

Integrating Feeling and Thinking Roles

The directors are responsible for the realization of the potential of the agency and must understand the importance of action and the mood in which the action is taken. Thus board function and power involve the integration of feeling roles (affections and emotions) and cognitive roles (thinking, exploring and problem-solving). To enjoy, realize and benefit from an agency's potential, the action must be founded upon sound planning and positive team application.

What Is Action?

To possess and demonstrate organized action involves an understanding of *what action is*, the levels of action and units of analysis. For example, Pfeffer (1982) identified three perspectives on action. In an assessment of the effectiveness of a voluntary agency board the following three types of actions are of prime importance. Action can be examined in terms of:

1. Prospective, intendedly rational and created action. Such action is planned and usually comprises part of a pre-determined structure of events. While the action begins the cycle of events, the action also is the initiator and, to a large extent, controls direction, intensity and inter-relatedness with other components of the organization or climate within the agency and society.

2. Externally-constrained or situationally-controlled action. Such action, which is a response to imposed conditions that are externally controlled, places constraints and even barriers on other types of action.

13

Such actions respond to situations that occur rather
than those planned.

3. Action that is almost random, an emerging process that
   is exploring possibilities. The action is internally
   initiated and is exploratory in an attempt to search
   out possibilities before planned action begins.

Individual and Organizational Action

Such perspectives of action can be analyzed in terms of the
individual (directors and employees) and the organization
(e.g. the voluntary agency). The three types of action can
be used to examine and assess what is happening within a
board in terms of each director and in terms of the performance of the board.
    Unfortunately, a fourth type of action occurs in
voluntary agency boards, that of totally random action,
where directors fail to update their information, fail to
read past minutes, ignore past decisions and actions and
vote with little foresight or understanding. Such
frustrations can be detrimental to the formation of a vital
and active board or to the maintenance of a hard-working and
competent president, executive and/or senior employees.

Examination of Quality and Abilities of Nominated Directors

In contrast, organized action depends on purposeful,
informed and vital directors, and in turn, such directors
bring about organized action. Such action must precede the
election or selection of officers. Organizational structures in modern Western societies emulate the underlying
principles of democracy through group participation and
decision-making, evident in the behaviour of members of
commissions, tribunals, committees, and in this case,
voluntary agency boards. A voluntary agency board comprises
a group of individuals elected to consider, deliberate and
finally take action upon designated or formulated matters
relating to defined areas of responsibility. Deliberate,
rational and planned action is a must in the selection of
the slate of officers and members of the board.
    A wise selection of candidates is essential; each
candidate should present a summary statement of the qualifications possessed, personal experience and accomplishments and what, if elected, the specific contributions will
be. A voluntary agency board is more viable and effective
with a small, vital and purposeful board than a large board
where meetings comprise a smorgasbord of attendees, some of
whom are poorly informed because of non-attendance, non-

commitment or non-contribution. Membership should normally be between nine and fifteen. Large boards are often hampered by lack of direction, by decisions determined by who attends the meeting, and further hampered by some members providing little or no contribution. Board membership size must be determined by a consideration of specific responsibilities for each board member, team-work contributions, organizational efficiency, and by the availability of appropriate and relevant candidates for office.

Membership Categories for Directors

One suggestion for the election of a balanced board of directors is that of membership categories for directors. The positions on the board are categorized to permit candidates to nominate according to interest or expertise. Such categories might include parents, professionals, business executives, persons with handicaps from within or outside the agency, media personnel and relevant minority groups. Another important category of board membership is that of employees. With an increasing awareness of the importance of sound employer-employee relationship, representation on the board of directors, apart from the attendance and participation of the senior employee(s), is necessary and beneficial. No doubt, a strict adherence to such rules might force the wider membership to seek out more appropriate candidates for office.

Controlling and Initiating Events

The efficiency of a voluntary agency board is directly related to the ability and competence of directors to control and initiate events by taking and creating intentional and rational action. Underlying factors for these conditions are:

1) organization of directors: committee structures:
   a) individual abilities and personal responsibilities;
   b) knowledge acquisition and demonstrated competencies;
   c) collective utilization of individual strengths;
   d) size and composition of board;
   e) positive feeling tone;
   f) brain power and accomplishments;
   g) essential committees.

2) decision-making:
   a) sequence of events in decision-making;
   b) problem-solving or challenge accomplishments;
   c) role of president;
   d) leadership;
   e) effective communication.
3) fiscal responsibility:
   a) budgeting;
   b) accountability;
   c) unit cost and cost effectiveness.
4) outreach activities:
   a) awards;
   b) interboard collaboration;
   c) national contribution and affiliation.
5) forward planning:
   a) past records and development;
   b) influence of government decisions;
   c) financial projections.
6) adaptive behaviour and risk-taking.

RESPONSIBLE AND CO-OPERATIVE ALLOCATION OF DUTIES AND TASKS

The organization of the directors on the board should be planned and involve individuals in a responsible and co-operative allocation of duties and tasks. Once a board's composition of members has been established, the first action is to designate individual responsibilities. One approach is the person-committee fit model (Kennett, 1984a). The utilization of the person-committee fit model encourages personal action by designating specific responsibility, through matching individual resource powers with the demands of the organization for which the board committee was established. Increased opportunities accrue because action is the first priority, a priority that leads to responsibility, knowledge acquisition, and flexibility in decision-making. Each person, because of a clear, designated responsibility, enjoys peer support and co-operation, and is motivated and encouraged to utilize personal strengths and interests. Although the model is being presented as one organized, rational approach for a voluntary agency board, the model has application in various domains of life such as business, education, and numerous professional associations.

Person-Committee Fit Model

The underlying premise of the person-committee fit model is founded on the belief that action is the beginning point, that action should create positive feeling tone and, finally, action brings about the thinking that rationalizes the action into a meaningful structure. Meaningful action relies on, at least, the recognition that;

1) all persons are individuals first who seek enjoyment, recognition, direct responsibility and delight in the personal utilization of strengths and competencies without the restriction of regular committee meetings and the frequent misuse of time and effort without achievement, and

2) accomplishment is the only evaluator of plans, proposals and programmes.

First Action

The prime task of directors is to support the work of those employed to assist clients. Initially a general conceptualization of agency function should be presented, the objectives provided, and a tour of the facilities and services taken to allow board members to know what they are about, to participate in the services they manage and to have personal contact with those they employ. Without these pre-requisites board members cannot bring relevance to their decision-making. Following this, individual members should meet, talk and participate in the functional areas of the organization by involvement with professionals, clients and support staff.

Second Action

The second action is to have members elect the areas of responsibility for involvement in a specified area, which will require the acquisition of competence to give expert advice and action during committee decision-making. This means the acceptance by each committee member of a cell of responsibility. Individual members bring unique characteristics and capabilities to the committee team and such strengths must be matched to appropriate tasks. Each member must have an assigned area of action and responsibility that supports personal growth, learning, self-evaluation, and improved human relations in working with permanent staff while seeking assistance from *significant others*, within and without the organization. Board members who fail to be committed to specific responsibilities are of no value to the voluntary agency board, and should either resign or, under peer pressure, reconsider their contribution. Many boards have a requirement regarding attendance at board meetings, with absence from three consecutive meetings leading to automatic resignation. Too many boards include members who remain inactive and non-productive, but still influence the direction of events by their voting power and arbitrary contribution to discussion at meetings. One solution is to motivate members to become involved and committed to successful ventures; those that do not become involved normally experience subtle peer pressure and find reasons why they are not seeking re-election.

Two-level Membership Participation

Members are also group members at two levels of committee membership, namely sub-committee and whole committee level. Group involvement is essential for an efficient committee requires interaction, feedback, competition, conflict, peer involvement and evaluation, maturity, and all the essential components, such as motivation and success, that tap the wealth of human resources and power possessed collectively by the committee. Goals and purposes need to be established as an ongoing process of events, integrating both long-term projects and specific tasks within the overall framework of doing and achieving rather than saying and planning. The purpose of the committee should be demonstrated not in lengthy board meetings but in the reported action of achievement, feelings of success that give positive support, and the thinking that places the action in correct perspective within the structure of the organization.

Utilization of Individual Strengths

Competent action will depend on the utilization of the strengths of individual members, the cohesiveness of team work, and the shared responsibilities of vital members as they encounter the process of collective decision and action.

Committees can improve their achievements by insistence on member participation, member training programmes, an understanding of collective decision-making, specialized individual competence, knowledge base, and sincere and meaningful commitment. According to Peters and Waterman (1982) a researcher concluded recently that *research effectiveness was inversely related to group size; assemble more than seven people and research effectiveness goes down.* Various big businesses, such as 3M and IBM, break into manageable units or divisions. Putting together a small, effective team to solve problems and ensure success has been carefully studied by Child (1977), who stated that once a group of ten to twelve commenced working together, the ability to see each other's contributions became readily acknowledged and utilized. Individual effectiveness became a collective strength for achievement. Working committees that take action need to be small, vital and productive. Thus, effective person-committee efficiencies depend on both the number of committee members, and on the election of appropriate members who must bring varied and different talents to the composition of the committee. All elected members must possess zeal, enthusiasm and vitality. A small committee of such members is a power-house for action; a larger committee of some members not possessing these essential components is a power-house that experiences too many short-circuits and blackouts!

DECISION MAKING

Vital and purposeful directors need to know how to improve decision-making and show that ingredient so often lacking in voluntary boards, the capacity to reach a decision by making up their minds and then taking action. Board directors must examine all the relevant facts, balance the probabilities and be decisive. Boards need guidance in rationalizing the process of decision-making. The order of events usually follows the pattern of:

1) defining the problem or challenge,
2) collecting and reviewing the facts,
3) proposing and examining alternatives,
4) seeking views of competent others,
5) reaching a decision,
6) evaluating the results and accomplishments and
7) developing a structure within which decisions are made.

Decision-making frequently revolves around problems and challenges. Boards encounter problems and seek possible solutions. Like individuals, boards sometimes fail to learn *the responses necessary for certain problems* (Dixon & Glover, 1984). That is, board members have developed a set pattern or rigid line of attack in relation to solving a problem, and fail to recognize that inappropriate responses are maintaining rather than solving the problem. Secondly, board directors may *not recognize that they already possess effective problem-solving responses* (Dixon & Glover, 1984). Often the answer is available but the inability to focus on the real issues prevents the utilization of response patterns that would solve and satisfy the challenges of a voluntary agency. Motivation is another factor in solving problems, while the last difficulty in solving problems is observed when effective problem-solving responses are hindered and blocked by emotional states such as excessive anxiety (Mendonca & Siess, 1976).

Problem-solving and Meeting Challenges

Problem-solving and meeting challenges occur regularly in voluntary boards, but often the board becomes a hindrance to progress as well as a brake on speedy decisions. Problem-solving and meeting challenges often involve finance where certainty of funding is never assured and where service needs increase, and professional staff are placed at risk of burn-out (see Chapter Twelve, Mendaglio and Swanson). Anxiety is a common experience of directors and difficult decisions are needed. In order to maintain excellent services, directors must rely on leadership and action by the president, who after meaningful consultation with senior employees and key board members, seeks the support of the board for recommendations and for decisions on behalf of the agency.

Such consultations and board support can be expedited by utilizing a committee structure that encourages participation, individual responsibility and efficient means of communication. Various diagrammatic representations are given in Figures 1 and 2 of the *Person-Committee Fit Model*. All have common elements in that a member is involved in at least two sub-committees of the selected committee matrix, and possesses a set, clearly defined individual responsibility that enables progress and development outside of the committee structure, and reinforcement and achievement from within the committee structure.

THE COMMITTEE MODEL

The model relies on the following stages of development:

1) establishment of administration (chairperson, deputy chairperson, and executive committee);
2) terms of reference;
3) specific goals to be achieved over a set time period;
4) allocation of each member to a cell-responsibility;
5) selection of sub-committee chairpersons;
6) development of team spirit in sub-committees;
7) focus on strengths and positive action;
8) acting, feeling and thinking - seeking and attaining solutions;
9) development of preventative strategies;
10) adaptation to powerful action through competence and flexibility.

FIGURE 1 PERSON-COMMITTEE FIT MODEL

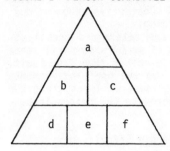

abc = Executive Committee
aef = Sub-Committee 1
bde = Sub-Committee 2
cdf = Sub-Committee 3

FIGURE 2 PROPOSED PROFESSIONAL ADVISORY COMMITTEE,
AUTISTIC CHILDREN'S ASSOCIATION OF NEW SOUTH WALES

- Areas of Responsibility -

	Development	Management	Finance	Committees
Early Intervention	a	b	c	Early Int. = a,b,c
Day Programmes (schools)	d	e	f	Day Prog. = d,e,f
Residential and Day Programmes (adults)	g	h	i	Res. & Day = g,h,i
	Dev. C'tee = a,d,g	Man. C'tee = b,e,h	Fin. C'tee = c,f,i	

Matching the Strengths of Members

Matching the strengths of committee members to specific tasks ensures increased interest, higher levels of achievement and develops positive self-concepts. At the same time, competition and conflict will be evident for they are integral parts of all human resource structures. Agreement and disagreement are ongoing experiences; maturity of response and action by all members determine the effectiveness of interaction, debate and decision. Such involvement permits clarification, reconsideration, political intrigue, manipulation, peer evaluation and persuasion of argument. Directors need to be alert to presentation and substance of argument that involve gimmickry. Showmanship, such as standing to make certain points or articulated expression, without supportive and substantive argument must be recognized and dealt with accordingly.

The workings of a committee are determined greatly by the leadership and the willingness of members to participate rather than procrastinate, to praise rather than find fault, and to insist on positive action. On the one hand, moments of debate may become heated and serious, while on the other hand, laughter and humour should permeate the proceedings.

Clarity of Purpose and Improving People Effectiveness

The success of a committee depends on the contributions of members and the clarity of purposeful action. The *person-committee fit* model is but the foundation for an organizational committee structure. The successful committee begins with such a foundation and adapts to the strengths of each committee member and harmonizes those individual strengths into an orchestration of action. As Peters and Waterman (1982) stated, *When we talk about improving people effectiveness, then, we mean giving people these kinds of opportunities to tap their own creative resources.* Cell-responsibility is the beginning of individual opportunities to act and action is the momentum that moves committees and voluntary agency boards into achievements (Kennett, 1984a).

STANDING COMMITTEES OF THE BOARD

Most voluntary agency boards require certain standing committees in order to administer efficiently the wide range of business that is directly their responsibility. Although names vary and differences in structure occur, such committees generally include the Executive Committee, the Finance Committee, the Professional Advisory Committee, the Fund-Raising Committee, the Staff Establishment and Salary Review Committee, and the Forward Planning Committee (to be discussed later in the chapter).

1. The Executive Committee

The essential overview and control of a voluntary agency board depends on the excellent functioning of a competent and active Executive Committee. This committee should not overpower the organization, but should facilitate the total co-ordination of all committees and ensure the smooth and efficient execution of regular board business. The degree of decision-making and the extent to which this committee determines policy and action is one which must be nurtured over a period of years, and through the establishment of confidence in the executive director. Membership usually involves office-bearers, such as the President (Chairperson), Associate Presidents (Vice Chairpersons), Treasurer, Secretary and those who chair standing committees and senior employee(s).

Initially, the Executive Committee on behalf of the board, has three major functions:

1) to maintain the efficient management of the total organization,
2) to make decisions that must be made between board meetings, and
3) to take responsibility for other decisions within the overall philosophy and forward plans of the agency.

Decisions made should be promptly reported to the board along with other business that should be well documented, supported by documentation and recommendation, and presented in order to provide clear communication and the opportunity to make sound decisions or comment.

The Executive Committee should co-ordinate and provide the harmony and tone of the board by expecting each member to bring forward recommendations from his or her particular committee and enable the President, through the Executive Committee, to have free discussion in reaching a consensus of opinion with resultant recommendations to the board. Sound and thorough preparation by the Executive Committee and President assists the board in acting efficiently and wisely. The Executive Committee should sift through the various issues, bring them into focus and present them for positive decision and action. Board meetings should be brisk, informative, and relevant because preparation for the board meeting encourages time to be used efficiently with accomplishments thus encouraging members to continue with their meaningful contributions.

2. The Finance Committee

The Finance Committee, chaired by the Treasurer and following consultation with the Director of Administration and the Accountant, should monitor the financial position of the agency, advise staff on what the board requires in terms of accounting information outside of that required for audit purposes, assist in forecasting future income, and provide monthly statements on unit income and expenditure. The provision of ongoing services continues only so long as finance is available. The Finance Committee alerts the board to financial dangers and needs.

3. The Professional Advisory Committee

The Professional Advisory Committee, following consultation with the Director of Professional Services or Executive Director, should advise the board on the professional activities of the agency in the following areas:

1) The pursuit of high standards of service through ongoing evaluation and accountability procedures;
2) The identification of needs and priorities with the establishment of at least one focal point in areas of quality and/or new direction;
3) The monitoring of trends in such areas as population, disability, educational, medical and social directions which could influence service provisions;
4) The production, maintenance, updating and contributions to professional publications and public relations.
5) The establishment of working parties on major professional issues, including position papers on disability, staff:consumer ratios, government services and subsidies, and various service areas pertaining to those of the agency.

This committee is an advisory committee that supports the senior professional staff, needs and services, and acts at board meetings as an informed group. The committee must keep close links with senior professionals. Co-operation is essential and this committee has the important task of maintaining and improving the relationship between professional staff and board directors. As with all functions of a board, the prime reason for existence is to give additional strength, support and encouragement to the professional staff who monitor and supply the essential services to individual clients. The directors should always be associated with the grass-roots, frontline action of the agency.

4. The Fund-Raising Committee

The Fund-Raising Committee, following consultation with the Director of Administration or senior Fund-Raising Officer, is responsible for the general planning and monitoring of fund-raising and associated public relations functions. The major responsibilities are:

1) The generation and evaluation of new fund-raising and public relations ideas;
2) The support of fund-raising staff in a consultant capacity;

3) The presentation of proposals, together with associated projected budgets, for new fund-raising/public relations schemes;
4) The monitoring of ongoing projects and their effectiveness;
5) The initiation of publicity to increase public awareness;
6) The recommendation of annual fund-raising budgets;
7) The provision of long-term fund-raising planning, including facilities and staff structures.

A dynamic, visible and competent professional service is the foundation for excellent financial stability through successful fund-raising ventures. Annual financial contributions rest upon the confidence engendered by the agency personnel. Major capital development depends upon endowments, government funding, contributions by public companies and on the recognition of a viable, achieving agency. Howe (1985) stated, *endowments and money for bricks and mortar depend on a conspicuously affluent and committed constituency, strong leadership, continuous planning and organization, enormous effort, and often the assistance of professional counsel.*

The directors have a vital role to play in the fund-raising business; they must be committed and the commitment must be demonstrated in their interest and involvement, their contributions, and their advocacy role in the community. *Nonprofit institutions that have achieved sound financial support are almost without exception those with trustees who are dedicated to the organization* (Howe, 1985).

Public relations and personal involvement by all associated with the agency are essential in sound fund-raising ventures. People reach people; people donate to people. Individuals give to individuals because of established confidence, respect, admiration and because they are known and associated with excellent service delivery.

5.   The Staff Establishment and Salary Review Committee

The Staff Establishment and Salary Review Committee is responsible for recommendation on new staff positions within the context of the total staff establishment and should make decisions on matters of salary adjustment and salary increases or promotion. In all cases a job description should be available, having been prepared by the appropriate senior officer and presented by this committee for board approval. Initially, the staff establishment needs to be fixed at a prescribed date, at which time the committee should review the total staff, salaries and positions in order to eliminate any inequities or duplication of services. When salary awards for others exist, employees

25

who qualify for a parallel position should be allocated salary accordingly; salary increases and increments are automatic. For other employees, the committee should have a regular date for six-monthly reviews.

The Staff Establishment and Salary Review Committee should be perceived as a forward decision and recommendation committee that ensures that employees receive salaries in accord with their competence and contribution. The committee can also act as an initial appeals committee to consider any staff problem that relates to working conditions, salaries and assigned tasks and responsibilities. The existence of such a committee encourages staff by the recognition that their well-being, conditions of work, salaries and work load and responsibilities are of the utmost importance in a well-managed voluntary agency.

The above standing committees of the board focus on essential areas of administration that must be considered if the board is to function efficiently. These specific areas are separated to draw attention to major areas of management and responsibility. The separation into discrete committees is on the basis of the needs of a large voluntary agency service. Each specific voluntary agency will modify and vary the actual way in which these areas of responsibility are managed; for example, in smaller voluntary agencies the above proposed committees will be decreased in number. In this instance, committees will take the responsibility of two or more of the areas designated for the above proposed committees. The important point is that these areas must be monitored, directed and decisions reached for the viability of a voluntary agency. Sometimes the committees involve staff representation.

AGENCY DEVELOPMENT

Procedure for Membership

The membership of a voluntary agency is usually open to all applicants, for individuals from all walks of life are encouraged to join, participate and contribute. Most agencies have a formal process of dealing with applications for membership. Usually, an application form is completed and, together with an accompanying membership fee payment, is received by the office of the agency. The board, at its regular meeting, receives the application and membership is conferred on the applicant. Reasons may exist to deny membership and the board is empowered to do so; however, in most cases, applicants are usually received without debate and welcomed into membership.

Eligibility

Most voluntary agencies permit, without any restrictions, all to enjoy membership. Parents, friends of clients and families, and employees are encouraged to become members. Some argue against the involvement of employees on the grounds of conflict of interest, but this is being perceived as more acceptable as the communicative and motivational factors are taken into account. More recently, clients have joined the membership and participated in board activities. Furthermore, an active campaign may be necessary to increase agency membership in order to increase the distribution of members, for example, among community and state leaders, commerce, legal and business leaders, members from various levels of management, government employees, professionals and university and college lecturers and professors and retirees. The strength of a voluntary agency board is the diversity and competence of the membership. All resources should be utilized in ensuring a dynamic and active membership.

Networking

The efficiency demonstrated by members of the board and their committees is extended and strengthened by the development of a network of communication and commitment, which utilizes the various strengths of the membership. Many activities and tasks can be accomplished by calling on members, who are often waiting to be asked and involved. The development of a sound network relies on contacts, personal approaches, encouragement and teamwork. For example, with a number of fund-raising events essential to the financial needs of an agency, the establishment of a network among the members allows for a contact person in the various suburbs or service units and their immediate community. The allocation for a set suburb of a specific responsibility to a single member allows for economies in time and expertise. The establishment of a local committee under the structure of the person-committee fit model can use a designated member to liaise with the central body (such as fund-raisers, administrators), the president and members of the board.

Successful Boards and Strong Action-orientated Presidents

Successful boards support strong action-orientated presidents to bring momentum to the voluntary agency and to maintain it by exciting employees, directors, government and private providers of finance. Risks must be taken, progress must be consolidated and strengthened for future development. Diverse opinions should be heeded only by contributors. Directors must possess an inner drive to perform and achieve by doing things. Too often, decisions are reached by a majority vote of directors whose only action for the month is raising their hand or uttering a *Yea* or *Nay*.

Quality of Management and Intensity of Motivation

The leadership of the board (the president aided by senior employees such as director of professional services and senior administrative officer) can increase the quality of management and thus increase the intensity of motivation in board members by:

1. Giving recognition and praise. Whenever a job is done well an expression of appreciation should be given. Extra effort or co-operation should warrant recognition. The top employees should have titles that give recognition to their contribution and seniority.
    Reward merit by appropriate action (bonus, salary review, awards for contributions).

2. Communicating. Fully informed board members and a fully informed general membership are pre-requisites for vital and purposeful action. Communication can occur in many ways including newsletters, information sheets, visits to facilities, attendance at major functions, reading board papers, and contributing to the action of the board.
    Board members should inform others, seek information from others, contribute, listen to others, and ensure that communication is based on an understanding of what is happening.

3. Delegating responsibility. This is a key concept in the person-committee fit model. Every board member must have clearly defined responsibilities, be encouraged to show initiative and purposeful thinking and be given opportunities to reach decisions.

4. Leadership. The president must, by example, show commitment, action and competencies that act as an example to board members, and as an inspiration to all involved in the voluntary agency board. The president must maintain the focus of decisions and activities on maximizing the opportunities for efficient programme delivery. This is only possible when close consultations occur between the president, the executive director or senior professional director. In a spirit

of co-operation and understanding through regular discussion these two persons provide the top leadership in the agency.

5. Goal Setting. Directors of the board need to have clearly defined goals and this includes establishing objectives, setting standards and having a plan of action. Information about achievements should be a major component in the communication network.

6. Interest and sincerity. Board members must provide the sincere interest that sustains an agency board and all employees by visiting the various facilities, knowing the key personnel, attending functions to show support, speaking with praise of accomplishments, and taking an interest in the clients.

7. Confidence. Directors of a voluntary agency board have a major responsibility to maintain co-operation and sound working conditions. Thus, they must show faith and trust in their employees and, taking nothing for granted, support their services and involvement by providing opportunities for self-development, higher qualifications and training, and conference participation.

8. Participation. Directors with vitality and purpose reach set goals by ensuring that co-operation and communication are ongoing components of daily activities. Thus, the board should invite discussion and ideas on major developments, provide a sense of belonging, and explain policy decisions to meetings of employees. On occasion, certain board members should be encouraged to participate in an in-house, in-service workshop.

9. Job Satisfaction. Job descriptions and responsibilities are devised in terms of perceived needs within the organization. They provide the basis upon which an individual is appointed. However, once a new member joins the team a degree of flexibility should prevail to tailor the job to the individual's talents, interests and concerns.
    Increasing job satisfaction is a major preventative method of eliminating frustrations and tensions, harnessing and maximizing the talents that exist and ensuring quality services by providing job satisfaction.

10. Total Purpose Through Effective Teamwork. The board and all components of the agency should have a total

purpose with a flow of information about services, providing harmony through increased co-operation and team-work. Each department has set responsibilities and duties that only have real meaning and effect when they assist other sections of the organization in terms of efficiency and understanding. Each organization is made up of individual purposes that must adapt and become a collective purpose based on the needs of the agency. As an integral part of the total organization, each individual needs to encourage other members to assure the establishment of a vital, effective team. Effective teamwork relies on a clear understanding of what the agency can do (according to the constitution) and what action is being taken to ensure regular evaluations of the philosophy and subsequent application of services.

11. Understanding of Constitution. An understanding of what the board can and cannot do, according to the constitution, frequently increases co-operation and decreases areas of conflict. Every agency needs to have copies of the current constitution available to their membership and filed in the *office* of each unit within the organization. All members should be encouraged to make constructive suggestions on improvements that can occur within the legal framework of the registered agency.

AGENCY AND COMMUNICATION

Collective Purpose and Communication Skills

Successful board action and strong leadership rely upon a meaningful and current philosophy that integrates goals through good communication. Sound communication skills encourage involvement, openness and consideration for others. A voluntary agency with a collective purpose and a cohesive organization is an organization that has taken action to:

1) identify and understand avenues for open communication;
2) strengthen one-to-one communication in various settings - interpersonal relations establish confidence and competence;
3) identify and explain specific roles and task assignments;
4) explain and demonstrate the range and variety of strategies, practices and programmes;

5) encourage regular meetings to facilitate under-
     standing of current challenges;
6) develop and reinforce participatory and leadership
     skills.

Effective Communication and the Total Community

Collective purpose relies on effective communication not
only among departments of the voluntary agency, but also
among all members and the total community of business and
government. Communication must involve:

1. The total membership. Regular newsletters, profes-
    sional information, interagency collaboration, new
    services, and up-dated reports of activities of the
    agency and board are essential.

2. Open administration and management. Records of minutes
    of board and other committee meetings should be avail-
    able at the central office for all members to consult.
    Financial records and full information on agency
    activities should be readily available.

3. Details on each major fund-raising project. Sound
    administration assures that all major fund-raising
    projects are given separate accounts, allocated a
    proportion of wages for those involved in terms of
    hours spent on such a project, the outlay of funds, the
    receipts, the viability of the project, the funds
    raised, and suggestions for next year if the project is
    judged a viable and profitable venture.

4. Full information of current financial standing.
    Regular and current appraisals of the financial
    standing of the agency are essential. Prevention of
    shortfalls and crisis management rely on current
    knowledge of what funds exist, what funds are assured,
    and deviations in the cashflow, failure of a fund-
    raising project, non-renewal of government subsidies or
    delays in grants.

5. Regular information and liaison with appropriate
    government departments. Regular information and
    meetings with appropriate government officers and
    members of parliament (including ministers) will ensure
    the flow of information, establish avenues of communic-
    ation, and provide easy access to important decision-
    makers when support or aid are needed. Meetings with
    senior government officers, parliamentarians, and
    government ministers should always include a report of

accomplishments and an acknowledgement of the important role played by government in that achievement.

6. <u>Annual report and supplementary documents.</u> The annual report is a major communication publication and should be of a professional and business-like standard. The contents of the annual report should include a message from a distinguished politician (appropriate minister or premier), a report by the president, a brief summary of developments including some pictures of any official openings of services or buildings, facilities or functions, a financial summary in accord with legal and audit requirements, and an acknowledgement of major donors including major subsidies from government. It should also include reports of accomplishments of major programme areas.

7. <u>Members' meetings other than the annual meeting.</u> At least one extraordinary members' meeting should be called between annual meetings for the purpose of bringing about important changes, discussing developments, and providing a forum for information on professional activities and fund-raising events. Such meetings are useful for discussing and making constitutional changes and alerting and gaining support from the membership on matters pertaining to changes in philosophy and services.

8. <u>Meeting-place of voluntary agency boards.</u> Often a voluntary agency board is located in a major centre but serves other regional centres. When this occurs, the board should schedule an occasional board meeting at the regional centre and invite members in that area to meet with the board prior to the board meeting.

9. <u>Speaking at service clubs.</u> A wise selection of speakers appropriate to service clubs should be made, a Speaker's Kit should be available and a specific project allocated for the consideration of the service club.

10. <u>Preparation of a booklet, Guidelines to Directors.</u> A board of vital and purposeful directors is a board that includes new directors on a regular basis. To ensure communication of past decisions, structure of the agency, job position descriptions, policies, and so on, a *Guidelines to Directors*, will not only ensure sound communication but minimize hours of fruitless activity and debate.

Communication: Information and Feedback

Communication involves the provision of information and subsequent feedback; communication also involves the enthusiasm that gains the involvement of others. The establishment of an efficient communication network includes key parents and personnel who have indicated their willingness to assist in specific areas/functions and whose strength will establish and maintain the ongoing activities.

Communication: Regular Evaluation of Finances

Essential and regular communication must occur in the area of finance. Fiscal responsibility is a board matter and directors must know the financial state of the agency through regular information on budget projections, book budgets, monthly estimates and actuals, cash flow and by giving the direction necessary to staff in terms of what the board requires rather than what the accountant wishes to provide. Frequently, directors rely, and justly so, on the accountant to provide the format for reporting the financial position, which may be from only one viewpoint: that of economy of accounting and audit purposes. In addition, board directors have an important role in seeking additional format of required accounts, such as a monthly summary of receipts and payments relating to designated units or service areas. The financial summary of each unit should include donations directly obtained by those in that unit, relevant subsidies, and all appropriate costs. Such efficient accounting directs attention to areas which may gain further assistance from government and private sources. Both employees and private supporters appreciate recognition of achievements and an association with a specific project. Thought should be given to what financial papers should come to the total board to eliminate confusion, while still providing the essential financial position. In general, directors need to know that on a monthly basis the agency is financially sound, that each unit is within projected budget, that specific units are in need of further subsidy submission to government and that other units could gain additional support, on a project basis, from representation to identified private sources.

Communication: Accountability

Accountability and security can only be gained from a regular monitoring of projected against actual budget, from the identification of problem areas and the seeking of additional government or private support, and from the efficiency of staff who, in conjunction with the accountant, are permitted to indicate to the board the accuracy of the monthly statement on their unit, encouraged to give suggestions and acknowledgement for their astute and dedicated awareness and effort in making their unit self-sufficient. This does not imply that professionals should be directly involved in fund-raising but that they must have a close association with the accounts, income and expenditure that dictate the extent and existence of services.

Communication: Outreach by Recognition of Special Achievements

Communication in the wider community of service may take the form of special awards. Special awards to contributors within the agency are essential in order to recognize and reward those special people who do so much in a voluntary capacity to assure excellent services. It is necessary to recognize those within the wider community who are involved in assisting developmentally handicapped persons and *at risk* individuals and families. This recognition may be gained by an annual award that is presented at a special luncheon/dinner or an invited speaker evening. One example, is that of the Autistic Association of New South Wales which annually selects a recipient for the Lorimer Dods Award for *excellence of work measured by State, National or International standards, a singularly outstanding contribution to the well-being of children, or dedication in the pursuit of performance well beyond the call of duty.*

Communication: Interagency Collaboration

Much is written about interagency collaboration (e.g., Elder & Magrab, 1980) with the focus on interagency professional collaboration and much less on interagency collaboration of boards of directors. Personnel and programmes may gain further momentum and support if directors of various agency boards recognize their common challenges, and gain one another's confidence. Far from being in competition with each other for resources, they can become a powerful influence on government decision-making through united and concerted presentations on major issues.

Communication: National and International Contributions

Finally, a board to be competent and alive must contribute to national and international bodies, in order to maximize and utilize available resources, to ensure the power of such bodies to make representation to governments. It is important to influence government and community policies and ensure that the most up-to-date techniques, strategies, and research findings are applied and gainfully implemented for the establishment of the most stimulating and rewarding environment for all who are at risk and, in particular, those who currently demonstrate a developmental handicap. Skills gained and improved competency of staff lead to greater accountability and increased training of clients. A similar statement applies to directors, who with increased skill and competence become more aware of accountability and of their need for increased training in order to ensure that the agency provides the best of service delivery.

Communication: Forward Planning

Forward planning focuses upon the links between past achievements, current provision of services and availability of funds, and the application of brain power to plan and predict what could and must be. The Forward Planning Committee should consist of all chairpersons of standing committees. For example, for the implementation of a three-to five year plan, strategies need to be developed. A forward planning document must include position papers aimed at ensuring government support, and maximizing community awareness and support, while allowing for changing attitudes and social conditions, and predicting, in terms of the agency contribution, the demand and types of service and facilities needed in future years. Financial projection may be determined by what must be achieved and how such achievements are financially possible. This may necessitate a week-end workshop with all key personnel - directors, parents, staff and identified and available media and corporate leaders. Every human resource should be sought in meeting the challenge of providing excellent services.

ADAPTIVE BEHAVIOUR

Adaptive behaviour has become a commonplace concept in the arena of service provisions for developmentally disabled individuals (Kennett, 1977, 1985). The total membership and all involved have, with efficiency and energy, contributed to effective delivery of services to enable individuals at risk to become more adaptive. In a similar fashion, directors must develop increased adaptive behaviour and with flexibility and fluency seek new solutions to old problems by pursuing new combinations and resolutions which remove obstacles (Kennett, 1984b). Risk-taking is an integral component of such action and must be encouraged and contained. New ideas and new solutions are as much the mandate of purposeful and vital directors as they are of professionals, fund-raising officers and administrators. Training, guidance, planned responsibility and involvement are foundation stones in the ongoing process of excellent service delivery.

SUMMARY

The management and administration of rehabilitation programmes is an essential component in the effective delivery of services for mental retardation. The board of a voluntary agency has major responsibilities, namely the power of decision-making, control over the direction of development and services, and the ultimate establishment of the conditions and opportunities that maintain and improve professional services. Quality voluntary agency boards consist of well-informed and competent directors who demonstrate purpose and vitality through their actions and accomplishments. Some of the major points are as follows:

1. Purposeful and vital directors acknowledge their prime purpose as the maintenance and improvement of professional services;
2. The effectiveness of a voluntary agency board depends on the calibre of elected directors and the working arrangement of the board.
3. The Person-Committee Fit model assists in developing an effective agency organization.
4. Problem-solving and meeting challenges is an integral component of board activities.
5. The president or chairperson is the figurehead, and a major motivator of action. He/she acts as both leader and consultant to ensure excellent services.
6. Intensity of motivation and quality of management involve recognition and praise, effective communication, delegation of responsibility, interest and sincerity, effective teamwork, a meaningful and current philosophy, and confidence.

A voluntary agency board depends on the calibre of the directors; people mean power to ensure vitality, purpose, enthusiasm, co-operation and action in order to develop personnel and programmes for the sake of excellent services. These afford, at best, each developmentally disabled individual a meaningful and fulfilling life within the community in which membership is enjoyed.

REFERENCES

Brown, R. I. & Hughson, E. A. (1980) *Training of the Developmentally Handicapped Adult*, C. C. Thomas, Springfield, Illinois.

Child, J. (1977) *Organization: A Guide to Problems and Practice*, Harper & Row, New York.

Dixon, D. N. & Glover, J. A. (1984) *Counseling: A Problem-Solving Approach*, John Wiley & Sons, New York.

Elder, J. O. & Magrab, P. R. (eds.) (1980) *Coordinating Services to Handicapped Children*, Paul H. Brookes, Baltimore.

Howe, F. (1985) 'What You Need to Know About Fund-Raising,' *Harvard Business Review*, March-April, 18-25.

Kennett, K. F. (1977) Adaptive Behaviour and its Measurement, in P. Mittler (ed.), *Research to Practice in Mental Retardation*, Vol. II, Education and Training, University Park Press, Baltimore.

Kennett, K. F. (1984a) 'The Person-Committee Fit: Effective Action and Responsible Decision-Making,' *College Student Journal*, 18(4), 355-358.

Kennett, K. F. (1984b) 'Creativity: An Educational Necessity in Modern Education,' *Education*, 105(1), 2-6.

Kennett, K. F. (1985) *Assessing Adaptive Behaviour and Social Competence in the Family and in Society*. Paper presented at the 7th World Congress of the International Association for the Scientific Study of Mental Deficiency, New Delhi.

Mendonca, J. D. & Siess, T. F. (1976) 'Counseling for Indecisiveness: Problem-Solving and Anxiety Management,' *Journal of Counseling Psychology*, 23, 339-347.

Peters, T. J. & Waterman, Jr., R. H. (1982) *In search of Excellence: Lessons from America's Best-Run Companies*, Harper & Row, New York.

Pfeffer, J. (1982) *Organizations and Organization Theory*, Pitman, Boston.

Chapter Three

MANAGEMENT AND ADMINISTRATION IN REHABILITATION: IMPACT ON
PROGRAMMES AND PERSONNEL

Roy I. Brown and Peter R. Johnson

Consumer Involvement

The nature of the responsibilities that have been described
in Chapter Two creates the atmosphere within an agency for
its development. Given a sound and effective decision-
making at board and management level we now look at some of
the issues relating to personnel and programmes. Staff must
have opportunities to make recommendations and be heard in
the process of board decision-making. It is also critical
to build in opportunities for advocacy by consumers in order
to ensure that desirable change occurs. They should have
direct input into a programme and may be appointed to a
board or advisory committee. In some agencies they are
encouraged to form their own committees, which not only
advise and comment on programme and sometimes on progress,
but also have direct links to other agency structures, such
as a residential services committee. Furthermore, managerial and programme changes must be measured in terms of
effectiveness, consistent with both consumer performance and
philosophy of the agency.

SERVICE DELIVERY

Evaluation of Programme Priorities

Just in the same way as we indicated in Volume 1 the need
for structured programmes, so we believe similar structures
are necessary for the management of an agency. One way of
examining philosophical and programme views in an agency is
to make use of simple tests such as that suggested by
Marlett and Hughson (1978) in their Value Priority Scale.
On this particular scale, individuals note their personal
priority by ranking 20 items in order of merit for the
development of a programme. They rank these same items in

terms of their appearance within the programme. Such a method can immediately show discrepancies between what staff think should happen, and what they think actually happens. It also provides an opportunity to compare and contrast the views of staff and to look at the views of board members and see how they vary, both between themselves and in relation to staff.

Figure 1, taken from the profile of a rural agency, demonstrates some variability between staff and board, but much greater variability intra staff and intra board. No common view was held and the board maintained the staff were incoherent and could not put into effect the board's philosophy. Yet examination of the board showed exactly the same problems amongst their own members. In this particular instance an opportunity was provided for counselling by an outside consultant. The aim was to enable the board and staff to establish effective communication channels and devise an efficient philosophy and programme base. It is here we see the role of the outside consultant to greatest effect, for the predominant role is as recorder and counsellor not as a director informing what should be done, but enabling staff and board to decide on a cohesive basis what they wish to be done.

Rehabilitation is changing continuously. New attitudes and ideas reflect not just new knowledge in the field of rehabilitation, but the changing political, social and economic climates within any particular country. If agencies are developed effectively individual staff views must be taken into account. It is important to encourage staff to think in abstract, long ranging terms rather than simply in terms of immediate needs and gratifications.

Integration of Programmes

Integration, at its best, takes place throughout and across vocational training programmes, home living and leisure training programmes. Unfortunately in planning for rehabilitation, we often fractionate programmes and force individuals in agencies to perform under different direction and different philosophies at different times of the day. It is quite possible for the staff in the day programme to believe in an individual's rehabilitation into a normalized environment while those in the evening programmes believe that this is impossible. Of course it may occur that people perform differently in different environments and this too must be taken into account. But we must know the philosophy and attitudes of staff involved and still attempt to produce integrated programming goals.

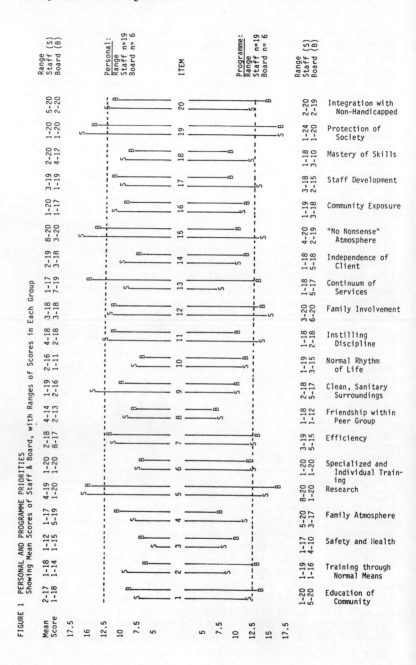

FIGURE 1 PERSONAL AND PROGRAMME PRIORITIES
Showing Mean Scores of Staff & Board, with Ranges of Scores in Each Group

This becomes even more difficult when the programmes are run by different agencies or different authorities, and argues for some comprehensive examination across agencies of their aims and directions. These issues should be discussed quite openly and clarified, both in terms of philosophy and the direction of programming, including the selection of staff. Unless staff support and adhere to the general philosophy (and, as they become increasingly involved in the agency, contribute to that philosophy) no strong programming integration can develop. As indicated in Volume 1, persons undergoing rehabilitation require a concise and structured programme where the goals are clear and do not conflict. Certainly in the early stages of programming, responses are not internalized and individuals are unable to make decisions of any great magnitude on their own. This must be supplied through a consistent and integrated programme structure.

The above perhaps has relevance to senior personnel and how they are given authority within an agency. Normally there are managers and directors of particular aspects of programme such as home living, vocational training and leisure time. However, it might be wiser to put someone in charge of a smaller number of clients and ensure that they are responsible for all aspects of the individual's training. Thus a director for 30 or 40 clients, dealing with home living, vocational and leisure time training, not only ensures one person is directing a consistent philosophy, but also creates an arrangement which provides links between staff, who have different functions, thus encouraging collaboration and discussion of individual programme planning.

This administrative procedure derives directly from the concept of the individual programme plan, because unless people are willing to meet over particular clients and devise specific, yet integrated, goals for different parts of the individual's programme, it is unlikely that reasonable training communication will take place.

There are other advantages. Staff have opportunities to move from one aspect of a programme to another while still remaining within the context of a similar philosophy, thus reducing stress and burnout. Furthermore, because there are a number of directors dealing comprehensively with a relatively small number of clients, different models can be employed for different types of clients or, indeed, differing programming may be examined with greater care at a demonstration level. The above is merely one example of the general service planning that needs to go on within any agency. Decisions are not made primarily for bureaucratic reasons. They are made for meeting the specific goals which must be set up within a particular philosophy for specific clients.

41

Roles and Characteristics of Successful Staff People

This argument leads naturally to the role and training of administrators and managers. For some while there have been arguments that individuals should be specifically trained for the role of administrator. If this means that they require skills in addition to those of programme personnel, one can accept this argument. But, the individual in the administrative role must know the business of rehabilitation. If the individual does not have knowledge of frontline involvement, then a number of problems arise. Rehabilitation cannot be run like a business in terms of a factory or industrial plant. Nor is the financial balancing of books of the same order as the balancing of books in production units, for *pay off* for the individual client in rehabilitation may be in ten or twenty years' time.

Progressive agencies may have many problems which include the *rumour mill* and stresses associated with burnout, as well as emergencies and the extreme views of a few staff members. There is also a wide range of personnel problems that interfere with the smooth running of an agency, and these often include problems connected with the individual's private life. These difficulties are not exceptions. They are normal events which occur in running an agency. If an administrator is going to deal with these concerns effectively, then he or she must have the skills of an experienced counsellor.

Leadership of staff is a critical aspect of agency performance. Within the demonstration field a variety of authors have produced a range of psychological and educational models or programmes which appear to work well in their own hands but less well in other people's. It may be that individuals are biased in presenting their own programmes, but it is probably true that identification with the programme concerned is of immense importance at an emotional level in producing effective results. Very few programmes written for the field deal with this inter-relationship. This espousing of the goals of the programme by those who are going to administer and instruct is essential. We suggest *an enthusiastic person with a bad programme is likely to have more success than a non-enthusiastic person with a good programme.* Although this statement may be rather extreme, it nevertheless illustrates the fact that we have paid little attention to the types of people who come into rehabilitation while paying considerable attention to the programme curricula. It is the integration between these two facets which is important and should be measured in assessing programme effectiveness.

What makes up an effective programme in the field? Social modelling, motivation and reinforcement practices are certainly the tools that must be understood and applied by administrators and managers as well as frontline staff. In selecting personnel, we have little firm knowledge of what constitutes staff effectiveness, and examination of studies looking at the prediction of positive educators has produced remarkably poor results. It is time to study the rehabilitation field carefully in terms of the activity and behaviour of team leaders and other senior personnel within the management structures.

One of the features that may be important is the flexibility of image that can be projected by a staff member, while at the same time recognizing the need for consistency of philosophy and goals of the agency. Beck-Ford and Brown (1984) have indicated a series of roles that an individual needs to go through in developing, defining and applying rehabilitation within the leisure time sphere. The recommendations made there apply to a number of other areas. A staff instructor may need to utilize the roles of controller, director, instigator, stimulator, educator advisor, observer and enabler (Avedon, 1974). The role an individual staff member takes depends on the handicapped person's maturity of response, knowledge and ability to internalize structure and ability to generate decision-making behaviour. One aspect of handicap, well known to us, is the variability of performance of disabled individuals. A staff member may need to change his or her role fairly frequently to adjust to the changes in behaviour and environment stress that occur for the individual client.

Administrators must also have a clear idea of the number of consumers they can know well. In our experience, when the clientele reaches more than about 100, the basis for decision-making about an individual becomes impersonal. It has to be based on the knowledge of other persons close to the individual, because the administrator does not have sufficient information from a personal point of view to make valued decisions.

Very often the administrator makes decisions relating to frontline issues based on written or oral information yet we know that when stress occurs it is visual information which tends to be more appropriate and effective in terms of a knowledge base for change. Thus in these situations the frontline personnel are critical in the decision-making process.

Agency Size

In western countries there have been cycles of growth and decline in relation to the size of operations. Although there has been a tendency to desegregate handicapped persons in recent years, there has also been an increase in bureaucracies within government services dealing with a wide

range of handicapping conditions. This has a number of
implications for the delivery and personalization of
service. It must be remembered that of all the types of
treatment, rehabilitation involves a personalized service
directed towards individualized goals. When it is a large
agency serving say more than 100 people, the senior
administrative and management personnel come to know:

a) little about the programme needs of the clients
    the agency serves,
b) little or nothing about the individual clients
    and, further, because they have no control over
    critical aspects of frontline liaison, they set up
    a bureaucratic administrative system which
    provides rigid rules of a written kind.

Thus inflexible rule-systems tend to be developed. It
is impossible to meet individual needs under these
circumstances. The possibility of making changes based on
demonstrated needs, the ideas of frontline staff or the
application of research findings is remote. One major
problem is that personnel in administration have little time
to update themselves in terms of advancing procedures and
knowledge. Some acceptable type of rotation system between
administrative and direct programme involvement might reduce
this concern.

Whelan and his colleagues (Whelan *et al.*, 1984) have
attempted to involve frontline staff in decision-making
processes, particularly in the area of research. There has
been some attempt in recent years to encourage frontline
staff to recommend research projects which might be of value
to frontline practitioners and clients. Whelan has made use
of this model to some considerable effect by organizing a
committee consisting of frontline workers to recommend
questions that they believe should be answered for the
well-being of agencies and clients. It is the research
worker's role to put these questions in a form and programme
practice that can obtain worthwhile answers. But as Blunden
and Evans (1984) point out, frontline staff find it very
difficult to accept evaluation at a research level, if this
results in implied criticism of their own activities. Once
again, some balance has to be found between impartial and
internal, yet informed, opinion. A bureaucracy that can
examine its own processes and recognize its own strengths
and weaknesses is one that is likely to encourage staff to
become involved in the same process.

Two other important moves which are encouraging the
modification of programmes are the development of an
advocacy system and, in North America particularly, the
development of self-advocacy through the People First

movement. Parents and advocacy systems have exerted tremendous pressures on special education systems (Sarason & Doris, 1979), and these have had detailed effects on programmes and programming at an individual level. It is also essential for college students of Rehabilitation Education to be able to apply the knowledge that they have learned. Furthermore, we must recognize that this does not represent the end of the educational process, and if Rehabilitation Education is to become a profession, then we must recognize the need for continuous education of all staff in all agencies. This means some ongoing negotiations and relationships between university and field units.

Funding, Philosophy and Programme Integrity

Voluntary societies must be able to generate funds in order to operate adequate programmes. Unfortunately, this task sometimes compromises their advocacy position and even raises accusations of exploitation of handicapped people.

For example, governments often provide voluntary agencies with funds for service delivery. Once this money is accepted, it becomes difficult for societies to lobby forcefully on behalf of their consumers since unsympathetic governments may eventually threaten to withdraw their financial contribution. Many members of the society will then be truly fearful of losing the service and some civil servants will believe that there are no further funds. Consequently, some voluntary societies will settle for the provision of a service of inferior quality rather than none at all. However, it is likely that a few people on both sides will be satisfied with poor quality because they believe that handicapped people are not worthy of more!

Vocational services are often especially poorly funded. Consequently, many agencies use a large proportion of the profit from their vocational enterprises to hire the supervisors and trainers. Workers are paid poor wages as in many North American sheltered workshops and British adult training centres. In other words, agency funds are generated by the productivity of handicapped workers who themselves remain impoverished. Thus a case can be made to support the notion that, in these instances, the consumers are exploited.

Unfortunately, this situation is currently worsening as agencies, under economic pressure to survive, must gain further subcontract work in order to have sufficient money to pay staff. The fact that community jobs are becoming less available means handicapped persons remain in training agencies longer, their stay occupied by more and more vocational work. This is the direct opposite of what is required in relation to training in social, home living and leisure time skills, and this represents the antithesis of normalization which rehabilitation philosophy has espoused (Brown, Bayer & MacFarlane, 1985). Governments, agencies, and the socially-concerned within the community should be made aware of this travesty of rehabilitation.

This situation is exacerbated by the government pensions often given to handicapped people. These provide a minimal standard of living, but are decreased by the amount recipients receive from employment. Clearly, this is a disincentive to independence as it punishes productivity. Pensions may represent charity in one of its worst forms, if they prevent the growth of independence and self respect in handicapped persons. Of course, a simple solution would be for governments to use these pension funds to support the vocational services, who could, in turn, pay meaningful wages to their handicapped workers (see Chapter Five). The fact that this approach is not taken is indicative of the prevailing devaluation of handicapped people.

An important issue for voluntary societies is the generation of operating funds which are free of government constraints and which do not further the devaluation of their consumers. One successful, if indirect, method is to maintain a high profile in the community, as this tends to produce a steady stream of donations and bequests which are occasionally large. In addition, some societies have used lotteries and bingo games with somewhat erratic success.

However, the most successful enterprises may be those in which voluntary societies have gone into business for themselves, and kept these activities separate from their service provision. For example, Thrift Village, Inc. (Value Village in Canada) is an American second-hand store chain which operates throughout western North America. In each community, this successful business attempts to negotiate a contract with a local voluntary society. In return for permission to use the society's name in the telephone solicitation of donations of used clothes and appliances, Thrift Village agrees to pay a substantial part of the profits in return. Because this is an extremely well-managed business, profit payments tend to be regular and substantial. An additional advantage of this particular kind of business, i.e. second-hand stores, is that it tends to do best in economic hard times.

Cost Effectiveness

It is not our intention to go into detail in the area of cost effectiveness except to say that it is a challenging and difficult issue (Conley, 1973). Most agencies do not keep costs in a very adequate manner and financial printouts are ill-understood by many staff. It is important that staff have an understanding of the basic costs of running a centre, not least because they can often suggest ways in which savings can be made. Unfortunately such decisions are often made at a bureaucratic level remote from the existing agency or, in any case, by senior management without major input from frontline staff. We argue for a better informed, more trained and sophisticated frontline staff who can participate in the decision-making process. In some of our consulting work, we have noticed that boards do not always regard their staff as professionally trained and able to make decisions. Yet this is a circular and self-defeating argument because if one wishes to improve an agency one must train and develop effective staff. They must then enter the decision-making process. This is one of the notoriously weaker areas of management, both in government and private agencies.

In the area of cost-effectiveness, decisions are very often made on the basis of short term gains. While one recognizes the managerial and financial reasons why this might be done, one is looking at long term objectives in the field of rehabilitation and therefore, although it may be less easy to cost the effects, the long term implications of decisions on an individual's lifestyle must be recognized and taken into account. At the present time, for example, many agencies are dealing with sub-contract work and from this work agencies make profits which enable them to hire their staff. However, as indicated, this also has a negative effect.

It has been argued that processes like normalization are cost effective. Although this might be true in mild cases of handicap, the more severe the disability, the greater expenditure that is incurred both in the short and in the long term. The arguments for such rehabilitation cannot be made on a monetary basis. The arguments must be made on a humanitarian basis, and on the effects of knowledge gained and applied. We recognize within our national defence budgets that expenditure of funds is a major item if it is deemed necessary for the country's protection. Likewise if the prevailing view is that rehabilitation is desirable for citizens, funding limits will not be imposed so as to terminate or reduce it.

Self-Help and Decision-Making

Self-help groups are an important aspect in the rehabilitation continuum and are discussed elsewhere, but the matching of programme offerings to student need must not be overlooked. One can now enter agencies where the handicapped individuals are essentially in charge of programming, and there is much freedom of choice but the amount of freedom can result in a loss of the structured basics of rehabilitation. For example, individuals who should be regularly walking and moving to ensure the exercise of damaged limbs, may receive no physiotherapy or training direction so that spasticity and muscle wastage is increased. There may be no opportunity to receive training in learning strategy and problem-solving techniques. Many handicapped persons are not in a position to make certain decisions or motivated enough to deal with particular questions of lifestyle.

EVERYDAY ETHICAL ISSUES

Confidentiality

In recent years, agencies have become much more aware of their moral obligations to their clients. In general terms, it is an essential move to ensure the various aspects of the individual's programme are carefully controlled and monitored. First, all new staff, board members and managers should be clearly aware of confidentiality of records. Information should not be passed from one agency to another without permission of the client or the client's sponsor, and such permission should always be in writing. The agency also has a responsibility to ensure that parents and clients are able to find out sufficient detail of the agency philosophy of functioning so that they feel comfortable in being part of the facility (whether, for example, the agency encourages advocacy), to act as a check, not only on its own programmes but on the needs of the individual.

Certain aspects of ethical procedures can be made a committee function. Such committees should in turn relate to the advisory committee or board of management of the agencies. We suggest that there are at least two committees to be seriously considered;

1)   an ethics committee;
2)   a therapeutic practices committee.

These two committees are crucial for the functioning of an agency. Some may argue that not all agencies carry out research. Nonetheless any worthwhile agency will encourage professionals to come in and use their agency on a research basis, although the agency must decide on the value of the research, for one aim is to stimulate and redirect the thinking and programming of the agency. Each of these committees will need to have clear guidelines and impartial and knowledgeable members.

The Ethics Committee is there to ensure that the practices carried out within the agency are not only ethical, but they are done in such a manner that individuals

48

have the right to withdraw or the right to know about them. It is not the role of this committee to say whether research is valid or invalid. This committee is there to ensure that the appropriate ethical care has been taken in the research or programme that is being carried out. Many ethics committees are concerned that names are kept out of research data, and have required, in some cases, that records be destroyed after research has been completed. We do not regard such practices as necessarily desirable. The retention of data can be important, particularly when one is considering the long term nature of rehabilitation. Indeed one might suggest, it is unethical to destroy data since others will have to re-collect it later. Rather than removing names from research data, the ethics committee might consider on what basis information is communicated. For example, in a recent study parents requested they be shown information reported by their child on the grounds it might help them to learn about their child and become more effective. This is laudable in itself, but individuals were adults who had passed on information in confidence. In this case the client's written and informed consent was necessary. Thus the basis on which information can be passed on needs to be clarified.

In addition, this committee should look at the nature of a specific research proposal. One of its aims should be to ensure that such research can be carried out, that not too much time is taken away from training. There is a need to ensure that research will be recorded in an effective manner so it can be utilized by the agency. For example, has the research proposer offered to provide feedback to the agency at the end of the study? Has the research worker clarified how long the study will take, both in terms of hours and in terms of total duration of the project?

We also believe that a *Therapeutic Practices Committee* is necessary. As we use behaviour modification and allied technology with individuals, there are conflicts at times between the use of various drug therapies and behavioural techniques. It is important for impartial committee members to assess the impact of any unusual or aversive techniques to be employed. However, impartial does not mean unknowledgeable. It means people who have no vested interest in whether a particular practice runs or not, but have sufficient knowledge to come to an informed opinion.

Staff-Consumer Relationships

One is often encouraged in professional training to distance oneself from one's client at a personal, social and emotional level. Such an approach was essentially derived from a medical model when concerns related to physical problems. The complexities of rehabilitation involving social, educational and psychological concerns, as well as the duration of the rehabilitation process, suggest much closer relations are likely to be engendered between professional staff and clients. If this is the case, then understanding and empathy are important but other emotions often occur and some bonding is likely to be made between staff and clients.

Staff may quite frequently act as substitute parents, relatives or friends. Sometimes the situation is made more complex by the fact that clients come from abusing families, or from situations where emotional support and social structure will be needed to provide motivators, not only for learning, but for the building of positive self image. Thus emotional ties are naturally likely to develop. These have to be mediated effectively to the advantage of clients since such relationships are for the benefit of the client only. Clients have to be helped to grow and move on. Care must be taken that the relationship does not become destructive or perceived by the client as a further failure.

ADVOCACY

The Politics of Lobbying

Advocacy, the act of pleading the cause of another person or group of persons, is a very important function of human service agencies. While this responsibility has been undertaken by many individuals over the years, it is only recently that agencies have become more sophisticated in dealing with the politics of power. Consequently, new methods of advocacy are becoming available to those people who wish to uphold the human rights of their handicapped friends and clients.

It is important to understand the relationship between the members of the society or agency and the government bodies concerned. Employees of agencies have limited value as advocates because they are often seen as being in a conflict of interest situation. In many circumstances, employees stand to benefit indirectly from the causes they are pleading. For example, if an agency obtains funds to set up a new group home, it is possible that the director will get a subsequent salary increase due to additional supervisory duties. Consequently, it is important that agencies have a volunteer wing who are perceived as altruistic. Voluntary societies already have this component, but other agencies must develop advisory committees if they are serious about personal and corporate advocacy.

As a general rule, employees of the agency should lobby members of the civil service. It is the elected representatives of the society who, along with the director, normally meet with MLAs (or MPs) and cabinet ministers. Issues are initially raised with line staff of the government (e.g. social workers), and then lobbying moves up through the hierarchy until the problem is resolved. This means that department heads of the society tend to meet with regional managers, while the executive director or equivalent, discusses issues up to the deputy minister level (senior civil servant). Often combined groups of staff and board members, such as a senior management committee, can be very effective in carrying the message to the seat of government using various kinds of political pressure.

SOME RULES FOR LOBBYISTS

1. Begin by planning strategy. Define your goal(s) and itemize an action plan. Review this plan on a regular basis because events can necessitate radical changes in your plans and even your goal.
2. In terms of government hierarchies on general matters, start at the bottom and only proceed to a higher level when you do not get satisfaction. However, as you proceed, keep the lower levels informed of your actions, as they may be able to bring some internal pressure to bear upon their seniors. Yet there are controversial issues which must be directed to senior personnel from the beginning. While responsive to government structure, do not let this force the same hierarchical model onto the agency staff model.
3. Never back the government into a corner, unless it is absolutely necessary. Always allow them the room to change their position gracefully.
4. Whenever you can legitimately make the government look good, reinforce and publicize their positive actions. The principles of learning do govern the behaviour of politicians.
5. Unless there is an upcoming election, do not waste time in cultivating the opposition. They are nearly always supportive but powerless. However, do keep them informed on important issues - just in case the government falls overnight!
6. Attack policies, programmes and laws, but never attack people unless it is absolutely necessary. Whenever possible let people know that they are doing a fine job, but with regard to that matter under discussion there may have been an error in judgment! Remember that personal antagonism can produce a lifelong enemy

of the society, and this can have a detrimental effect on the lives of handicapped people.

7. Consider employing a paid lobbyist at the seat of government. In North America, this is a respectable position, and the role of the incumbent is well understood by politicians. Paid lobbyists arrange frequent meetings with government officials, present the views of their employers, and make sure that the concerns of the society maintain a high profile among the politicians.

8. Do not be afraid to call in political debts. Some members of voluntary societies are members of political parties, have friends who are politicians, and may have even worked on electoral campaigns. Occasionally, a telephone call to a friend in the government can produce a much quicker solution than lobbying through the system.

9. Use the media in an escalating manner. On any particular issue, begin with human interest stories, move to policy concerns, and finally discuss the role of the government. Be prepared to be misquoted and misrepresented, for sometimes members of the press are less concerned with veracity than with an interesting article.

10. However distressing it is to be the target of hostile comments and attacks against your personal integrity, try to evaluate these in a positive way. They are often a sign that the other side is feeling the pressure of your campaign and in fact, you are making progress.

CONCLUSION

In developing this chapter we have attempted to look at the needs for programming for individual clients and its reflection on staff and management structure and board interest. A few general conclusions have been reached.

1. Consumers should be involved in the development of programmes which are to serve them.

2. There must be evaluation of philosophy and programme priorities which enable conflicts and agreements between the various parties to be examined carefully and resolved effectively, if necessary, with the help of an outside consultant.

3. There needs to be integration of programmes for each individual consumer. This has major impact on the development of services.

4. One effect of individualization of programming is the need to keep numbers small. A model is suggested to

ensure that a team leader or unit manager can direct a small team of personnel covering integrated programmes for a small number of individuals.

5. It is argued that little work has been carried out on the nature of the interaction between personnel and programme delivery. The need for enthusiastic and knowledgeable staff, who believe in the programme they are administering, is essential.

6. Personnel must be sufficiently well trained that they can carry out different roles which match the needs of particular clients. This versatility assumes a wide knowledge and a period of detailed training and experience for each staff member.

7. Concerns are expressed over agency size and the impact this has on individual clients. It is suggested that the development of modern bureaucracies limits the possibilities for the development of individual programme planning and makes it difficult to provide adjustments to dramatic or gradual shifts in programme needs. Some suggestions are made for coping with this situation.

8. The need to develop funds, which can overcome concerns relating to the selection of particular vocational work in adult rehabilitation is stressed. Rehabilitation means more than vocational work and there is some danger in present society that abuses may follow the development of poor economic circumstances in society as a whole.

9. Comment is provided on the nature of cost effectiveness and long term goals.

10. Ethical issues are discussed together with the importance of ensuring adequate monitoring groups within agencies to ensure that development in terms of research can take place, without subordinating the needs of individual clients.

11. A section is provided on the politics of lobbying and a series of rules are suggested to help an agency develop an effective programme of communication and development in its relations with government and allied systems.

REFERENCES

Avedon, E. M. (1974) *Therapeutic Recreation Services. An Applied Behavioral Science Approach*, Prentice-Hall, New Jersey.

Beck-Ford, V. & Brown, R. I. (in collaboration with C. Rolf & M. Gillberry) (1984) *Leisure Training and Rehabilitation: A Program Manual*, C. C. Thomas, Springfield, Illinois.

Blunden, R. & Evans, G. (1984) 'A Collaborative Approach to Evaluation,' *Journal of Practical Approaches to Developmental Handicap, 8*(2), 14-18.

Brown, R. I., Bayer, M. B. & MacFarlane, C. (1985) *Rehabilitation Programs Study*, National Welfare Grants, Health and Welfare Canada, Project 4558-29-4.

Conley, R. W. (1973) *The Economics of Mental Retardation*, Johns Hopkins University Press, Baltimore.

Marlett, N. J. & Hughson, E. A. (1978) *Rehabilitation Programs Manual*, Vocational and Rehabilitation Research Institute, Calgary, Canada.

Sarason, S. B. & Doris, J. (1979) *Educational Handicap, Public Policy and Social History*, Free Press, New York.

Whelan, E., Speake, B. & Strickland, B. (1984) 'Action Research - Working with Adult Training Centres in Britain,' in R. I. Brown (ed.), *Integrated Programmes for Handicapped Adolescents and Adults*, Croom Helm, Beckenham, Kent.

Chapter Four

MANAGING CHANGE IN REHABILITATION SERVICES

Aldred H. Neufeldt

INTRODUCTION

This chapter is about change. Its intent is to summarize
some of the major dynamics of the change process as they
affect human services of various kinds, and to set out ten
steps through which holistic change may be accomplished.
The data base underlying the ideas set out is derived in
part from such seminal writings as Trist (1978), Schon
(1971), Ackoff and Emery (1972), in part from discussions
about these matters in the context of a graduate seminar on
human service organizations at York University, Canada, but
in good measure the ideas reflect nearly 20 years of
involvement in the introduction of change processes into
various human service systems (mental health, mental
retardation and others) and an examination of the impact of
forces of change on both public and private, large and small
systems (Neufeldt, 1983a; Neufeldt et al., 1983; National
Institute of Mental Retardation, 1982). A fundamental
assumption throughout is that change in our human service
systems is not only inevitable, it is desirable - not for
the sake of change itself, but for reasons of improved
service quality for persons with disability. In short, this
chapter is about creating a desirable future and the means
that leaders in the field can employ to shape the direction
of future services in more rather than less positive
directions.

THE INCREASING RATE OF CHANGE

The word *change* is an ever present part of our vocabulary.
We *make change* (money), or change clothes, trains or jobs.
Property *changes hands* and political leaders change. In all
these examples there is an implied underlying constancy.
While change takes place, it does so in the context of a

55

larger continuity - a mere substitution of money, clothes or leaders. There may be a change of form, but not of substance. Chevalier at York University talks about this as marginal change.

Periodically *change* is used in another sense - the significant altering or transforming of a given situation. When a large and once stable institution is phased down and out of existence, or when the fundamental premises on the basis of which human services exist are altered, something more substantial is occurring. The entire focus and approach to the service becomes transformed reflecting the new understanding of purpose. There is a change of both substance and form.

It is this second class of change that is of central interest in this chapter. The former reflects the marginal adjustments any organization must make on a day-to-day or year-to-year basis. The astute manager will anticipate adjustments to be made and introduce appropriate processes to accomplish these changes. Such adjustments are the hallmark of an effectively run organization. However, few human service leaders learn how to anticipate let alone implement a process of substantial change. Most organizations wishing to transform themselves find it exceedingly difficult to find a leader with the kind of background and experience in whom they can trust. Yet it is just this more substantial change process for which we need to become more prepared.

A convincing case can be made for the assertion that there has been more substantial change within the human services in the past three decades than in all of the previous century, and that such change is likely to continue with increasing tempo. Universally available rehabilitation services provided the first major impetus. This was followed by changes in quality of human services as quantity increased. Large scale services are devolving to smaller scale more dispersed service forms. Twenty years ago, for example, the developmental disability field was characterized essentially by large residential institutions. A few group homes had been developed (15 in all of Canada in 1966), as had the beginnings of sheltered workshops and some special schools. The prevailing assumption in much of the professional community was that the more severely mentally handicapped individuals were not capable of learning despite the fact that Tizard (1964) in England had demonstrated the contrary some 15 years earlier.

By 1978 more than 450 group homes and apartments had been developed in Canada along with a large number of sheltered and semi-sheltered work options and special education programmes across Canada many of which were beginning to appear in regular public schools. Between 1966 and 1978 something obviously had changed. These changes are not abating. Ten years ago in the province of Ontario a *group home* was so defined that a residence housing up to 50 persons could qualify. In 1985 legislation is being passed which will define as an *institution* any cluster of disabled individuals living together totalling more than 10 persons (even two group homes side by side).

These changes represent the tip of a much larger change in assumption about the nature of rehabilitation. In part this is a reflection of societal changes over human rights. Concern for *the person* is taking its place alongside concern for the *service*. In part there is a shift from *information centred* to *criterion centred* decision-making.

Those of us involved with the mental retardation movement in the early 1970's were acutely conscious of the fact that the basic knowledge was available which should have made it possible for mentally handicapped persons to live much more self-sufficient lives, but that the mainstream of the service system including most institutions of higher learning, who were training future service personnel, were ignoring this information. A prevailing assumption up to that time in all the human service systems was that if you gave a responsible professional the right information then the right decisions would be made. Yet, this obviously was not happening. Given this failure Canada's National Institute on Mental Retardation (NIMR) examined the decision theory equation ($d = f (i \times c)$, i.e. the decision made is a function of the information one has and the criterion used), and decided it was time to challenge the criteria used by policy makers, professionals and others. NIMR's starting point was to introduce the normalization principle (Wolfensberger, 1972), a developmental model and related concepts in a nation-wide campaign of training events, seminars, films and conferences. Focussing attention on values and first principles galvanized action immediately.

It is predictable that changes in human service will continue at an accelerated rate for the same reasons that the rate of change in all of society is also increasing. Aided by computer and information processing technology the half-life of knowledge continually is being reduced. Whereas we once were dependent on a few *authoritative sources* for our ideas about what *state of the art* programming was like, today there are many sources of such information. When communication is almost as easy between Jerusalem and Toronto as between Toronto and Calgary it becomes a simple matter to transmit information on innovations of merit from one place to another.

But simply having knowledge of innovations will not promote the necessary change above. For example, computer technology is remarkably seductive, tempting one to believe that more and better refined information is what is really important. Apart from an appreciation of values important to achieving qualitatively sound human services, we also need to have knowledge about the dynamics of change. The remainder of this chapter deals with the nature of the change process and steps which can be taken by a human service leader to ensure changes undertaken are sound.

FIGURE 1   STAGES IN THE ADOPTION OF CHANGE AS RELATED TO THE AMOUNT OF ENERGY REQUIRED TO ACHIEVE THAT CHANGE

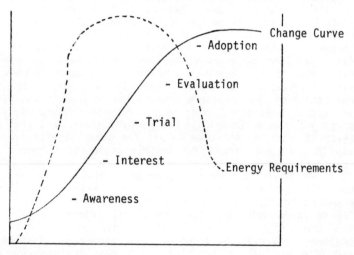

DYNAMICS OF CHANGE

The essence of creating change is to persuade others that they should adopt a new set of ideas and ways of behaving. A sizeable body of literature has been published on how knowledge becomes disseminated and used by others (e.g. Havelock, 1971). Most individuals, groups and systems proceed through a number of stages in first considering and then eventually adopting a new innovation (see Figure 1). One first must be made aware of an innovation and its potential merits before interest can be obtained. A tremendous amount of energy is required from the initiator of the change process to create such awareness and interest, largely because most of us are so caught up in our busy and closed systems that we have little time for anything that does not immediately fit within our immediate frame of reference (and innovations rarely do). If sufficient interest can be obtained then the innovation may be tried, and if tried then evaluated. Finally, if all these tests are passed the innovation may be adopted. At each stage along the way there inevitably is a great temptation to abandon the process, largely because of the forces of the *status quo* (what Schon calls *dynamic conservatism*). The early strategy, therefore, has to be to capture a small number of persons who are the *early adopters*. As a growing number of individuals and groups begin accepting the innovation then the initial energy input, to induce people to try the change, can be reduced. For most individuals that point is reached when they are persuaded to try the innovation. As any good salesperson will testify, a battle is at least half won if a potential customer will test their product. So too with innovations in the human service field.

To infuse new and improved ways of doing things into our human service systems is more difficult than it sounds. This is equally true whether the reasons for change are essentially positive (i.e. conditions improve for everyone involved) or negative (i.e. one group may suffer in the process). Many examples might be used to illustrate the kinds of problems experienced, both large and small. Sometimes the underlying dynamics involved are most easily seen in large-scale ventures simply because the underlying issues are thrown into bold relief. Two examples follow;

Vignette 1: The Challenge of Phasing Down Large Residential Institutions.

Late last century and the first half of this one, it was commonly believed that the best means of providing services for persons with a number of different problems (e.g. mental retardation, psychiatric problems) was to create large residential care settings. A number of rationales justified the practice (Wolfensberger, 1974). When first begun in the late Nineteenth Century such residential centres were to provide a place where expert resources could be assembled to provide the best form of treatment in the most effective manner. These original rationales were lost at the turn of the century with pressures from the eugenics movement. Despite continuing efforts by a minority of professionals to maintain humane conditions programmes deteriorated to the point that, in essence, these residential facilities became large warehouses filled with humanity having little prospect of release.

Such institutions usually were built in communities some distance away from urban centres. These smaller communities inevitably became highly dependent on them for employment, particularly as the institutions grew in size. One particular psychiatric institution serves as an example (Neufeldt, 1983b). Located in a small prairie community of 7,000 people, the institution at one time (early 1950's) housed 2,000 individuals. In the mid-1960's it employed approximately 1,200 personnel at the time. The next largest employer in town employed 40.

To initiate change in such a system raises all manner of anxieties. Chambers of commerce and town councils fear change because of possible adverse economic effects. Ward staff and professionals who have carved out clear and predictable ways of relating to each other, as well as to administration and inmates, fear change because of uncertainty as to their new roles even when continuing employment is assured. Administrative personnel whose status and power have been derived from the size of staff supervised and size of budget administered find change traumatizing because neither large bureaucracy nor buildings may be as central as once thought. Even larger and distant empires become threatened. A host of specialized businesses and industries have grown up over the years with residential institutions as their primary market; e.g. manufacturers of institutional furniture and institutional clothing, drug suppliers, food services providers, and architectural firms that specialize in the design and building of institutions. Each one of these stake holders inevitably raise barriers to the proposed changes. From within their own vested interest, all have legitimate concerns. Few bother to determine whether the concerns and needs of service users, the institution's residents, will be better served through the proposed changes. In fact the existing stake holders inevitably argue that substantial change is not required at all. What is needed, they say, are some marginal adjustments involving greater expenditure of funds to improve the building, or staff salaries, or increase the number of staff.

Vignette 2: The Challenge of Developing a New High Quality Service.

Putting into place a new and unique service is no less complicated than phasing out an antiquated one. To illustrate some of the underlying dynamics consider some of the barriers confronted by the Canadian Association for the Mentally Retarded (CAMR) in introducing its 'Plan for the 70's', the development of comprehensive community service systems (National Institute on Mental Retardation, 1982). The nature of the situation at the outset has already been alluded to. More than 200,000 persons classified as mentally retarded were incarcerated in institutions at the time involving an expenditure estimated to be one billion dollars in 1972. There were only a very limited number of community services, and those that existed frequently exhibited the same low expectations of their clientele as was typified in the larger residential institutions. The overall goal was to cause the development of comprehensive community based services systems. As a means to an end CAMR promoted the development of a series of ComServ Experimental and Demonstration (E and D) projects. A plan and guidelines were developed and published by NIMR (1973), and a detailed strategy of change was embarked upon by the Institute.

An 'awareness raising campaign' was launched by introducing parent groups, professionals and policy makers to the normalization principle, to concepts of what was meant by 'comprehensive community services,' and to notions of advocacy. A number of incentives were used to attract and engage both individuals and groups within all target populations in a testing process. At the individual level we adopted a strategy of training future trainers. After any given training event individuals were identified who the organizers felt showed the best prospects of both under-standing the issues involved and had the potential ability to lead discussion groups and/or lead practice evaluation teams (as in the NIMR PASS training programmes designed to teach people the nuances of the normalization principle). From team leader one might progress to assistant trainer and, eventually, a trainer role. This inexpensive approach not only proved to broaden the Institute's outreach capacity, it generated sound understanding and intense commitment to both the cause and underlying concepts. At the larger group level we offered the possibility of becoming designated as a 'National ComServ Experimental and Demonstration Project'. Again, intense interest was gained in many of the provinces of Canada.

Support for the ComServ Plan emerged in particular from parents with children who were under-served in the community, idealistic young service personnel, and mentally handicapped persons themselves. Policy makers in three provinces quickly embraced the basic concepts - Quebec, Saskatchewan, and Alberta. All three had just elected new governments at the time, each committed to introducing new and progressive legislation on behalf of mentally handicapped persons. Others followed with varying degrees of speed.

However, in even the most progressive of provinces points of resistance quickly became evident. In particular professionals and leaders of existing service systems (both institutional and community) tended to be very cautious about whether the normalization principle really contributed anything substantially new, and at times were extremely hostile. Orientation sessions not infrequently led to intense and sometimes heated exchanges. Parents of children in institutions also expressed great concern about whether their son or daughter might have to come out and how they might be taken care of, and agencies concerned with other disabilities began showing signs of resistance, in particular it seemed because too much attention was being paid to mental retardation. As a result policy and political leaders in the most progressive provinces began backtracking on some of their promises.

The 'E and D' Projects became the targets of additional forms of resistance. The federal government which at one time had committed itself to 10 such projects revised its agreement down to two. Within the two provinces where 'E and D' Projects were established the amounts of money which had been promised to help establish the desired range of community services seemed to disappear. A not undesirable form of unofficial competition arose between the 'E and D' region and other regions within both of the provinces designated, Alberta and Quebec. However, the net result tended to see somewhat greater amounts of funding and attention within the province devoted to regions other than the E and D region. Other forms of resistance also appeared (National Institute on Mental Retardation, 1982). This kind of experience, of course, is typical of that experienced by pilot programmes. It is of interest to note that once the five-year E and D period was over, these pressures were removed from the designated regions, more funding became available, and policy restrictions on the regions were lightened in both provinces.

BARRIERS TO CHANGE

The examples described above are but two of many which might be used to illustrate underlying dynamics involved in changing from one service form to another. Small organizations go through very similar experiences as large ones. The only essential difference seems to be one of time - a smaller organization can be changed more rapidly than a large one. Resistance derives from a number of sources.

1. <u>The Nature of Systems</u>. The nature of systems themselves contribute substantially. Schon (1971) proposed a concept of *dynamic conservatism* to explain this phenomenon, the seemingly active attempt on the part of systems of all kinds to avoid change. A related concept is that of *system lethargy*, the notion that systems are fundamentally lazy, finding it easier to avoid making any attempt to change than exert the effort required to adapt. As pointed out in another article (Neufeldt, 1983a), the most salient issues being debated today in a field such as mental health are essentially the same as those of 20 years ago. It somehow is much easier to debate an issue than to begin making changes in the system.

2.   The Nature of Disciplines. A second barrier to change
     is inherent in the nature of the disciplines involved
     with providing human services. In part, the very
     process of being trained to be a professional leads one
     to think of oneself as competent. Over time this
     competence tends to become dated, particularly when a
     substantial change in values or outlook occurs. But,
     by continuing to lean on a mythology of competence it
     is easy to avoid looking at alternative ways of doing
     things.
         A second type of problem stems from the way in
     which the various human service disciplines view the
     problems experienced by their clients. Each discipline
     views the client and his/her problem from its own point
     of view and tends not to think of other points of view.
     Yet the people who come to our doors for assistance do
     not arrive in disciplinary form. A person with
     cerebral palsy does not simply come with that one
     condition, yet there is a tendency for the members of
     each discipline to see essentially only the condition
     from their own frame of reference.

3.   Stress, Uncertainty and Other Red Flags. The volum-
     inous recent literature on stress points out that no
     change takes place without some stress. Changing one
     job for another leads to a stress response no matter
     whether the reason for change is an opportunity for
     advancement or a firing. As a corollary, it also is
     true that the longer a person has been in the same job
     the harder it is to change and the more stressful the
     change on the person: so too with organizations. A
     system in which employees are used to the regular
     infusion of new ideas or change is likely to exhibit
     less by way of stress response to an innovation than
     one in which little change has occurred over time.
         Marginal change is likely to be accommodated more
     easily than *substantial* change. For example, replacing
     typewriters with word processors in an office is easier
     to accomplish than changing the organization's purpose
     from one which offers a segregated, static vocational
     day programme to one which actively seeks to train
     disabled clientele in the regular work place. Both
     types of change are likely to cause stress and anxiety,
     and both could lead to extensive resistance on the part
     of staff if not handled well. But the one is rela-
     tively more easy to accomplish than the other in good
     measure because the change outcome has more reference
     points with what already exists. A word processor,
     after all, in many respects is an enhanced typewriter.
     In contrast the very essence of a shift from a static

to dynamic organization and from segregated to integrated services shifts almost all the reference points
simultaneously.

A substantial shift in reference points leads to a
further personal response - *uncertainty*. Both individuals and organizations evolve stable habit patterns
unique to themselves some of which are well recognized,
but many of which are implicit and go unrecognized.
Anyone who has moved from one agency to another, or
even from one regional office to another in the same
organization, has discovered that the local understanding of *how things are done* varies considerably from
place to place. When the essential purpose of the
organization changes, and when points of reference
disappear, then traditional habit patterns may not only
be unhelpful, they may be counterproductive. A problem
experienced in many large residential institutions, for
example, is that managers at all levels of the organization are used to maintaining the status quo within a
very rigid hierarchical structure. When a directive is
handed down from ministerial level that services are to
change in a substantial way (e.g. that large residential institutions are to become more consistent with
the new philosophies and principles by reforming
programme practices and phasing down in size), the
existing habit patterns of institutional management
make a positive and effective response next to impossible. Almost invariably new management and leadership
is required. At the same time some (but not all) of
the existing management, given a change in situation
and the opportunity to orient themselves anew, can
become very adept within the community service system.
Most participants in institutional change processes suffer from an acute sense of uncertainty about job
security, their future, and their own competence.
Given such uncertainty it is not surprising that
resistance occurs. Rumours arise in large numbers,
sometimes suggesting that the institution will be
closed overnight and sometimes suggesting that everything will return to normal (i.e. no change). It is of
interest to note that a similar phenomenon occurs in
towns and cities experiencing either too rapid a growth
or the demise of their sustaining industry (Neufeldt et
al., 1983).
Along with rumours, mythologies materialize. Such
myths may either help or hinder the change process. A
new leader introducing change into an organization will
quickly come to be viewed as weak or strong, reasonable
or unreasonable, etc. by persons wishing to maintain
the existing status. Within limits the experienced

leader will take advantage of the mythology of strength to assist the change process. Similarly, an organization acting as a change agent (such as the NIMR did in the 1970's, and as do the boards and staff heading up innovative new programmes) will evolve myths of competence. Whatever the myths, once established they are very difficult to alter - particularly those myths which are damaging to the intent and course of change. For this reason it becomes critical to select a leadership and staff to introduce a proposed change process who are likely to engender positive rather than negative mythologies.

Uncertainty, mythologies and stress seem to be not only a consequence but an essential precondition to change. Without a loosening of attachment to a former way of doing things, change will not happen. Their presence in a situation also means that an opportunity exists which, if not taken advantage of, will likely make future change all the more difficult. A new director of an agency usually has only a few months (three to six) in which to initiate change processes before the turbulence associated with the change subsides and coalesces into a shell of resistance. Beginning changes too quickly runs the risk of changes proposed being ill considered and failing on that account; but, waiting too long means that intended changes will be extremely difficult to institute. The time frame for relatively structured systems is much shorter than that for fluid, open systems. In introducing the 'ComServ E and D' projects and related Plan for the 70's the investigators felt they had approximately three years in which to gain sufficient momentum for change before forces opposing the goals would begin to slow the process.

A final potential problem is that if feelings of uncertainty are allowed to persist too long a vacuum in moral leadership will be created. Some organizations gain a reputation of being unmanageable. This happens when a succession of attempts have been made to introduce change processes, usually with different purposes in mind, each serving to increase the sense of uncertainty more, and successively diminishing existing adaptive patterns, and none of the change efforts lasting long enough to have any enduring effects. A vacuum of principle and morality emerges in such a context leading to behaviour on the part of some staff which is normally unacceptable, but which in such a situation goes unreported for long periods of time. Such a vacuum can only be overcome through an intense and lengthy infusion of positive and purposeful energy. Leadership perceived as temporary will not engender the kind of confidence required of staff to change their situation, most of whom deplore the existing state of affairs.

TEN STEPS TO CHANGE

Getting from where we are now to where we would like to be is a little more complex than it appears on the surface as is apparent from previous sections. First, it presumes we know where we are now and how we got there. Second, it presumes we know where we would like to be. Both presumptions are at best only partly true in most organizations. But knowing where we are going is only the first part of the battle. We still have to get there. While a sizeable amount has been written in the near past about desirable human service values which should frame the goal, and even more has been written about planning, little has been written about the implementation process. This section presents a number of rules of thumb to fill that gap.

Step 1: Frame the Issue. From the confusing mass of concerns present in a situation requiring change, there is a need to isolate the key issues that a change process should address. Problems that immediately are brought to the fore include such issues as insufficient resources, lack of responsibility or role clarity. But these types of issues usually mask the real problems. The fundamental issue to be addressed in human services usually relates in some way to the clientele being served. Framing the issue in terms of client needs has a way of allowing one to see issues of funding adequacy, personnel role and training needs, and so on in a new light.

The author is involved at present in assisting with the planning for and development of appropriate services for disabled children and adults in the Middle East. The region involved has a large refugee population, it is under military occupation, which means that a variety of tensions exist between the occupiers and the occupied and, consequently, it also has no central authority responsible either for the development and implementation of standards of service nor is there a taxation base for such services in the usual sense. Yet, over 30 agencies concerned about disability have appeared in this environment usually with the assistance of external funding sources. All have poor continuing funding bases, staff are generally inadequately paid and inadequately trained, and co-ordination between the agencies is largely non-existent. Many of these problems are recognized by some of the more foresightful agency leaders, but there is a uniform tendency to blame their current political status for their problems. While the occupation complicates all matters, and is the central issue from a political point of view, it is not the central issue from a service point of view. There is considerable doubt that any of the service problems would disappear even if the political situation were resolved. What we are trying to do is to encourage the service providers to reframe their concerns in terms of the needs of handicapped persons. Once this is done the other issues, including problems associated with military occupation, can be dealt with as they affect service development. In fact there is reason to believe that the universal concern towards persons with disabilities in today's climate would enable the development of sound services even in a troublesome political context.

Step 2: Values Clarification. Having framed the issues it is critical to identify the fundamental values inherent in addressing the issue. Values to be considered occur in at least three levels of interest. First, there are those values denoting support to or nurturance of the clients of the organization. Desirable values for human service users are denoted by key words such as *growth opportunities, dignity, quality of life* and *continuity*. A philosophy that *the customer is always right* is equally as applicable in the human service sector as it is in department stores.

But, there are secondary order values as well. What do we want for the personnel of an organization? Presumably we wish to have working conditions which are interesting and challenging, salaries which meet at least basic minimum needs, and opportunities for personal development.

Finally, at the level of organization as a whole some value expectations also come into play. Society, for example, expects the organization to be cost effective, and to economize.

The process of values clarification identifies relevant values at all three levels. Then, the relative relationships of these values to each other need to be established. Which values are primary? What trade-offs will be tolerated? Does one, for instance, trade-off individualized programming opportunities for cost? There frequently is an argument one should do so; yet, it is not at all clear that one needs to. Giving thought to these and other similar issues prior to the beginning of a change process is critical because changing practices repeatedly will test conclusions reached.

Stage 3. Image the Future. Knowing where we are now, how we got there and what is fundamentally important by way of values, we are then in a position to project a mental image

67

of the ideal state of affairs we would like to see. Some feel this is to be wasted exercise. Why should one pay attention to what cannot be achieved in any event is the question. People holding such views fail to grasp the essential purpose of future imaging. They tend to be so much caught up in the day-to-day problem of fighting the proverbial alligators that there is little opportunity to find out how to *drain the swamp*. By projecting an image of the future one gains a sense of the nature of the swamp we are in. The design itself is not utopian. It can be improved upon. What we are seeking is not an ideal system, but an ideal seeking system - a situation in which everyone involved in creating an image of the future not only asks *what would our service look and be like if we had our way*, they also ask *how can we keep improving the situation*.

The power of such futures imagery might be illustrated by example. Consider changes in mental health systems with those in mental retardation/developmental disability systems. Compared to 20 years ago the mental health system today has made some changes; but, in many respects is also very much the same (Neufeldt, 1983a). However, without question the mental retardation system has changed drastically. Whereas in mental health there still is ongoing debate on whether or not *mental hospitals* are needed, a debate that has continued for over 20 years, that no longer is a significant issue in mental retardation. Virtually every governmental domain in Canada is working at depopulating its large mental retardation facilities and introducing alternative programmes which, in turn, continue to evolve. I believe that in good measure this was due to NIMR's ability to set out a clear image, to friends and skeptics of change alike, as to what a normalizing, dignifying, developmentally oriented network of services would look like.

Great pains were taken in Canada during the early to mid-1970's by the National Institute on Mental Retardation to develop slide presentations which combined many different experiences to paint a picture of what *might be* if all such experiences were brought together. Interpretive tours to both *good* and *bad* programmes helped give people a mental picture of the possible and the undesirable. A Plan with guiding principles was devised that, if followed, would assist leaders (consumers, service providers, policy makers) to move towards an improved form of service which would begin approximating the ideal (National Institute on Mental Retardation, 1973).

Step 4. Clarify Interests. If a desired change is to be adopted the interests of groups involved must be satisfied. Corresponding to the values framework described above one can identify at least three sets of interests - those of the service users, those of the personnel involved either directly or indirectly in providing the services, and those of the organization itself (as represented by management or a board). Each may be subdivided further depending on the complexity of organization and/or environment. All three groups have a legitimate stake in the outcome of any change process. The concerns of all three may also vary from each other. So, for example, job security usually looms large as a critical interest of employees whereas getting more effective work for money spent is that of management. Both of these in turn can mitigate against the kind of improved services which users are looking for. Even when both organization leaders and staff members are pursuing the question of improving services for users their interests may differ substantially.

A change agent, or manager of change, should know the interests of all parties. A process should be introduced to clarify such interests, either through one-to-one discussions or group sessions. Because service users' views are usually least well represented, particular attention needs to be given to ensuring that these are well obtained. Indeed, given the relative power of the other groups in the situation an astute manager of change processes will use this as an opportunity to enable service users to gain some greater power over the state of affairs through the use of forceful advocates or similar means.

Having appraised the interests of the various players, a *currently perceived choice chart* might be set up. Such a chart itemizes the various interests for each of the groups involved, and against these summarizes the costs and benefits (plus, minus, no effect) for each plausible outcome. A five or seven point scale usually is most beneficial (e.g. very negative effect, minimally negative effect, no effect, minimally positive effect, very positive effect). From such a chart the change agent will be able to make some judgments both of the benefits as well as the costs of undertaking proposed changes to each group. Interests do not have to be equally well satisfied for a change to be accepted. The prime movers of the change process (usually either service users or management) are of course concerned that their own interests are well satisfied. They hope that personnel will agree. But as long as personnel interests are met in at least a minimally acceptable way it is likely that the proposed change will be adopted. For example, if management wishes to introduce equipment to automate the office more, service users are little affected and therefore will not display much interest. But office personnel will be greatly affected. Therefore, it is critical that their interests are met at least adequately, otherwise the equipment is likely to malfunction, productivity is likely to slow down rather than speed up, etc. Similarly, in introducing changes in form of service it is imperative that personnel see the advantages for service users. At the same time, personnel need to feel that the proposed changes will, at a minimum, not affect them adversely. Preferably the changes will also be seen by personnel as giving them new opportunities they did not have before.

Step 5. Maximize Legitimacy. Introducing change is a process in persuasion as much as anything else. To help convince people that the proposed new programme directions are not dangerous and, while different, offer significant advantages (at least to one of the interest groups) their legitimacy must be maximized. All parties must be able to appreciate and agree that what is said to be the case is in fact the case. The best way to ensure this is to develop objective criteria by which judgments can be made.

This was worked at in a number of ways within the mental retardation movement. At a client programme level functional assessment tools were adopted to demonstrate objective growth in learning skills. From the espoused values about the worth and dignity of the individual, and the nature of services we wished to see in place, a variety of principles were derived - normalization, developmental orientation, continuity of experience, comprehensiveness, and so on. These became yardsticks against which judgments of the adequacy of the service system could be made. To enhance interest, these principles became the cornerstone of 12 criteria against which nationally designated 'E and D' projects were to be established (National Institute on Mental Retardation, 1973). To judge the quality of a given programme or service system Wolfensberger and Glenn (1975) devised the PASS system of programme evaluation. Based on the normalization principle, this tool provided an empirical reference point against which the adequacy of existing services could be judged. These and similar techniques became important vehicles to ensure that objective and verifiable reference points could be established and tabulated against the decisions made, thus measuring whether or not services are improving, whether clients are better off, and whether personnel are suffering or flourishing.

Step 6. Invent Options. When first exposed to a projected change most people are somewhat skeptical. Some people see proposed ideals as impossible to attain, others spot weaknesses in them. In either case it is important for persons likely to be involved in a proposed change process (whether user, staff member or manager) to assume some ownership of the potential changes. The best way of accomplishing this is to invite as many as possible of each group to participate in an invention process. Every situation has its own uniqueness. This means that values, and the ideals associated with those values, must be translated into the context of that situation's environment. While principles remain the same, the specifics of their implementation will and should differ. An infant stimulation programme in a densely populated metropolitan area will not work the same way as in a sparsely populated rural area. Vocational rehabilitation solutions in an area of heavy industry should be different from one with light industry. Invention of options as to how principles may be best translated into a local context is not only a desirable, it is a necessity. The worst mistakes are made when insufficient thought has been given to such an invention process. Lesser developed countries, for example, too frequently accept solutions from more developed countries without critical thought leading, in turn, to the introduction of solutions which are unworkable or make matters worse. In one North African country several years ago I was shown a grand new, large rehabilitation centre, identical in detail to one in Northern Europe. The building meant to house up to 300 clients was empty. There was not sufficient electricity for the plant. Personnel had not been trained to provide the necessary services. And so that plant gradually decayed. Similar, if less obvious, mistakes are made within more developed countries. By inviting all parties to participate in a process of invention - not of the fundamental values and principles, but of how such values/principles might be implemented - one not only ensures the least probable mistakes being made, one also invites a commitment to change.

Step 7. Building Relationships. The leadership of a change process is particularly vulnerable to potential isolation. If the leader has any capability at all, she or he is likely to be respected, feared, loved and hated all at once. This also means that the leaders rarely will have someone from whom unbiased advice can be routinely obtained.

To ensure that the leader does not make decisions which are counter-productive, processes need to be introduced which ensure the leader is well informed of the various diverging views and forces. Fischer, a noted Harvard expert on negotiating strategies, proposes an ACBD principle - *Always Consult Before Deciding*. An active and continuing consultation process is critical to ensure open lines of communication. Not only does this help to ensure that there are no surprises, it also demonstrates to all parties that even if the ultimate decision is not exactly what had been

71

hoped for, at least the decision maker cared enough to consider alternative options.

Step 8. Empower all Sectors. The introduction of change will work best if in the process all groups (including the least powerful) find themselves with more power over their own destiny once the change is completed. Change which leads to disenfranchisement and a lessened ability to determine one's own fate can only create problems in the long run. This is most graphically illustrated in the context of disability work in the Middle East. Both occupier and occupied care passionately about their own peoplehood. Both are also becoming increasingly conscious of the needs of disabled people in their midst, with the occupiers having more resource advantages. When, as some-times happens, the occupation authorities offer to help the occupied they are resisted - for understandable reasons. Apart from whatever political implications there would be in such *collaboration* (a bad word in that context), demon-strating to one's occupiers a lack of knowledge would also illustrate one's powerlessness. Therefore, an essential by-product of the consultation process is to provide the occupied people with a knowledge base and model services that are at least as good as, if not better than, those of the occupiers. When this happens, then each party will have something to offer the other on the basis of mutual respect.

The same analog holds within a human service. The most powerless group in human services usually are either the service users or frontline staff. If office personnel can feel a growth in power, competence and equality vis-a-vis their supervisors, then introduction of new office automa-tion equipment will be perceived as less a threat and more an opportunity. If service users are given the opportunity to participate in the decision-making processes around their own treatment goals, then there is much greater likelihood that service plans will be followed through. If frontline personnel are given the opportunity to help redesign the ways in which they deliver the services, service quality is likely to improve. In all cases individuals involved will feel a sense of control over their own destiny which leads to greater personal satisfaction.

Step 9. Communicate/Listen. Problems with uncertainty, personal feelings of vulnerability and rumours were described earlier. To combat these tendencies improved techniques of communication must be developed. *Active listening* approaches where the leader deliberately tests what is being said during a consultation process should be standard practice. A useful step for a larger organization embarking on a major change process is to set up a permanent, credible continuing source of information pertaining to both purposes and nature of change being pursued. People affected by the change need to have the opportunity to have their questions answered by such a credible source without fear of intimidation. A related step is to enable representative members of the various interests to obtain information from others who have had similar change experiences, to provide some glimpse of not only the future, but also the adaptation processes required. Organized interpretive visits to places which already have experienced similar changes are useful for this purpose. Finally, special support counselling assistance may be required for persons having particular difficulty adjusting to the changes.

Step 10. Commit Carefully. The final rule of thumb when introducing a change process is to ensure that any commitments made by the leader(s) are carefully thought out. This does not mean that much time needs to elapse; rather, that decisions made are congruent in a number of ways. A decision must be congruent with the values being espoused as embodying the change process, otherwise the integrity of the purpose of change comes into question. Decisions need to be congruent with each other, otherwise a host of administrative problems will arise which will ultimately undermine the thrust of the change. Finally, decisions made must be congruent with the nature and character of the decision maker. All leaders have their own personal style. If decisions are made which appear inconsistent with that style, confusions will appear and again aggravate all the other uncertainties present in a changing environment. By *committing carefully* the manager of the change process is both modelling how a congruent approach to bridging values and practice is possible in a changing situation, and providing a symbol of constancy to others caught up in the flux of change.

CONCLUSION

Participating in a process which leads to substantial change can be a gratifying and exciting experience. It can also be frustrating, painful and depressing. Which experience one has depends in good measure on quality of leadership. Poor quality leadership in an organization going through a change process results in that organization being adrift, subject to external forces which appear capricious and unpredictable. While the organization may change, the experience to participants is unsatisfying and full of frustration. Good quality leadership in the same organization, facing the same circumstances, leads to much more positive experiences for all concerned. The manager who exercises good quality leadership knows and understands the dynamics of and potential barriers to change.

Even though the degrees of freedom available to good and poor leaders are the same, the good leader will make much more effective use of available resources than the poor one. The power to create change depends on a leader's ability to frame essential issues, to grasp the values inherent in creating change, and to project an image of the future which provides participants the possibility of gaining a measure of improvement in their lives. The ten steps to change outlined in the final section above summarize the essential means that, if followed, will enable the leader of a human service agency to manage change effectively and to the satisfaction of service users, agency personnel and the leader alike.

REFERENCES

Ackoff, R. L. & Emery, F. E. (1972) *On Purposeful Systems,* Aldine Atherton, Chicago.

Havelock, R. G. (1973) *Planning for Innovation Through Dissemination and Utilization of Knowledge*, Institute for Social Research, University of Michigan, Ann Arbor.

Neufeldt, A. H. (1983a) 'Searching for New Directions in Mental Health Services ... For New Times,' *Canada's Mental Health,* 20-24.

Neufeldt, A. H. (1983b) 'Social Design Implications Related to Mental Disability,' in *Design and Technology of Barrier Free Environments for Disabled Persons*, Health and Welfare Canada, Ottawa.

Neufeldt, A. H., Doherty, G., & Finkelstein, J. (1983) 'Myths and Realities: A Comparative Examination of the Impact of 'Boom' and 'Bust' Conditions on the Quality of Life,' *Canadian Journal of Community Mental Health,* (special supplement No. 1), 81-92.

National Institute on Mental Retardation (1973) *A Plan for Comprehensive Community Services for the Developmentally Handicapped, and Guidelines*, Downsview, Ontario.

National Institute on Mental Retardation (1982) *Experimenting with Social Change,* Downsview, Ontario.

Schon, D. (1971) *Beyond the Stable State,* Temple Smith, London.

Tizard, J. (1964) *Community Services for the Mentally Handicapped*, Oxford University Press, London.

Trist, E. L. (1978) *New Directions of Hope,* University of Glasgow, John Madge Memorial Lecture, Glasgow.

Wolfensberger, W. (1972) *The Principle of Normalization in Human Services*, National Institute on Mental Retardation, Toronto.

Wolfensberger, W. (1974) *The Origin and Nature of Our Institutional Models*, Centre on Human Policy, Syracuse, New York.

Wolfensberger, W. & Glenn, L. (1975) *Program Analysis of Service Systems (PASS)*, National Institute on Mental Retardation, Toronto.

Chapter Five

IMPACT OF AND ALTERNATES TO CORPORATE BUSINESS MODELS IN
REHABILITATION

Nancy J. Marlett

INTRODUCTION

As rehabilitation programmes mature and become systematized,
policies and routines generate and guide much of our
behaviour. Policies or themes organize and describe our
experience, predict consequences and lead us to control the
conditions influencing our lives (Kouzes & Mico, 1979;
Schon, 1971; Bandler & Grinder, 1975).

Schon (1971) emphasizes the power of theories stating
it is misleading even to distinguish between social systems
and theories for the social system is the embodiment of its
theory, and the theory is the conceptual dimension of the
social system. Kuhn (1962) maintains that paradigms affect
the very structure of human communities and the transform-
ation of paradigms is necessary for social change.

There are many ways to identify and understand our
underlying policies or models (Brown, 1984). Marlett and
Hughson, (1979) described a number of practical role models
within rehabilitation which have an impact on the mutuality
of interactions between staff and clients. These models
involved dependent models (medical, detention, sheltered
care, parental and trustee), transition models (instruction
and counselling) and independent models of work, home and
leisure.

Service Delivery Models

Marlett (1984) proposed five major service delivery models
that have a marked impact on service delivery, staff roles
and programme standards.

1. Welfare Models are based on the belief that people
    share responsibility for one another. This shared
    responsibility, implemented through government policies

76

and programmes, carries with it the obligation to ensure an equitable distribution to those who cannot provide for themselves. This basic tenet has resulted in services that:

1) are offered to those who can prove eligibility: disabled persons are more likely to be accorded support by virtue of their assumed incompetence;
2) provide subsistence level of support: persons receiving support are expected to adopt a charity posture, i.e. persons who are receiving support/- day programmes, must be seen to be compliant, content and grateful; and
3) are maintained as long as status (i.e. incompetence) can be verified.

In rehabilitation this has been reflected in our residential services, both large and small, that provide basic support in an economic, and equitable (i.e. standardized) fashion. Many of our day programmes reflect the same basis.

2. Professional Models have emerged from two distinct foundations - medicine and education, but they are essentially the same in their intervention basis. The belief in a cure or remediation contrasts dramatically with social welfare models which support the status quo. Professionals who are charged with the responsibility of preparing persons for re-entry into society assume high status because they are going to salvage people and make them productive members of society.

This is the most prevalent model in rehabilitation with both educational and medical orientations producing modern, comprehensive and professional institutions. The impact of these settings has been more pervasive than many of our earlier welfare institutions because of their high status and business profile.

3. Self Help Models The essence of self help is a philosophy of human dignity, social cooperation, mutual responsibility and mutual aid. While this is not a new phenomenon, the current self help movement reflects a growing impatience among people who are disenchanted with current social programmes and services or who feel isolated from the mainstream of social life. Self help parent groups of the 50's were a reaction against the social welfare models of institutionalization just as, more recently, self help groups of disabled adults are a reaction against the loss of personal power experienced in professional models.

4. <u>Social Action</u> Social action is based on the belief that problems emerge in society because of the scarcity of power and resources. Those with power and wealth are loath to share it. Devalued groups are created and maintained by those in power to justify the imbalance. Disabled persons, single parents, visible minorities and elderly people are not providers, but users and therefore not worthy of power or wealth. In the U.S. the movement toward redressing the balance of power (the civil rights movements of blacks, women, gays and disabled) has been dramatic in impact, yet often short lived. The Canadian and British approach to social action emulates the vitality of the American models but is balanced by a natural conciliatory nature - creating a social action dialogue and planned change process wherein disabled consumers assert their basic rights to supports that will enable full membership in society.

5. <u>Partnership Models</u> - We have currently a limited number of models which are attempting to augment the empowering aspects of self help and social action with power of professional skills. The difficulty of blending peer support with professional services appears to be extraordinarily difficult, as is the emerging role of the able bodied professional in a self help base.

BUSINESS MODELS

The impact of these service delivery models on the person with a disability, service providers and society at large is great, but there is an overriding business orientation emerging within rehabilitation systems. One needs therefore to understand the context of management models and theories and how these affect interactions with disabled persons. Management theories or approaches set out what is assumed to be true, and within that, what the organization is, what it does, and what it values (Schon, 1971). Rehabilitation services have been altered by an increasing reliance on covert management beliefs. If we are to be in control of our evolution as a service, we must understand the paradigm shifts that have changed the values we hold as central.

Reasons for Adopting Business Based Organizational Structures

In the early stages of development most human service organizations are built on a small group's direct and personalized response to individual needs. However, there are a number of powerful influences which transform small informal services into large formal structures.

here is an overwhelming pull in North America toward *growth economy*. It is believed that if a service is needed or good it will grow. Small human services are often treated as immature - not quite developed. Most volunteer services move into a staffing pattern as the needs become legitimized, and with the appointment of staff comes the need for ongoing funding. This need for funding causes organizations to emulate and aspire to the characteristics which funders value. Because funding bodies, in almost every situation, are bureaucracies, small groups quickly emulate hierarchical structures.

The subtle pressure on agencies to become large and structured occurs not only from government funders. The same situation appears to be occurring currently with voluntary sector funding. United Way, a comprehensive voluntary funding system throughout North America which has traditionally supported small, informal solutions is gradually and subtly moving small self help solutions into voluntary organizations based on business practices under the guise of assisting voluntary organizations to become more attractive to corporate business supporters of United Way.

The attraction of business structures is predicated on the assumption that we can increase efficiency through specializing resources and creating organizational structures dedicated to the accomplishment of stated organizational goals. This is in keeping with governments' drive to public accountability. Health and Welfare systems - the two main funders of rehabilitation programmes, are the two largest businesses in North America. One can understand the need for the appearance of accountability even though the costs to the taxpayer escalate with staffing structures dedicated to bureaucratic checks and balances.

Not only do voluntary organizations emulate government, the actual presence of government in rehabilitation is considerable. Governments still run many rehabilitation services directly, e.g. institutions, client management. In other situations where funding comes from one governmental source the structural and functional linkages cause a blurring of the voluntary/government functions. Still other rehabilitation services are the result of a service shift from government to the community sector. These agencies are essentially agents of government - deliverers of public funded services who operate under the permissive aegis of token boards of directors (Salamon, 1983). This has been particularly popular with deinstitutionalization - transferring persons from large state facilities to *community operated mini institutions* (for mentally handicapped, emotionally disturbed, brain injured persons). These *community boards* deflect public attention away from government, and yet the boards often discover they have the responsibility but no discretionary power related to funding, admissions or standards of care.

Impact of Technocratic Bureaucracies in Rehabilitation

The pressure on service agencies to emulate business also occurs because of a poor self concept as capable organizations. Because many rehabilitation services reside in the voluntary sector, they have inherited the reputation of being poor and weak sisters in the eyes of the *management authorities*. Many corporate leaders (as well as their scholarly admirers) direct the same combination of charity, pity and patronization toward voluntary sector administrators that society does to less fortunate segments of our communities (Heller & Van Til, 1983). There exists a strong belief that manufacturing has outperformed service because it has for a long time thought technocratically and managerially about its functions, whereas service has lagged because it has thought humanistically.

There is an assumption that the technocratic bureaucracy of business and industry is the ideal paradigm for all realms of organized effort. Management principles, and organizational development, have evolved from this model (Trist, 1977).

Bureaucratic structures (Weber, 1948) consist of the following:

1. A hierarchy of super ordinated authority relationships.
2. Administrative rules to guide organizational tasks.
3. Decision-making procedures adhering to technical and legal rules.
4. Administrative behaviour based on the maintenance of files and records.
5. Administration as a vocation.

Within most of our rehabilitation settings we have used technocratic bureaucracies to implement a professional model and thus end up with obstacles that reflect both (Marlett, 1985). We have adopted systems to provide services that have subtle and seductive powers.

Weber (1968) says of bureaucracies:

The formal characteristics of bureaucracy tend to neutralize the otherwise personal, emotional, irrational, and other often political behaviour for the bureaucracy offers job security and compensation along with a high degree of certainty of expectations and

*performance in return for the relinquishment of
independence and autonomy of action.*

Weber (1968), Denhardt (1981), and others suggest that
these organizational characteristics foster certain rigid
and autocratic personality types. Diamond (1984) further
proposes that the bureaucratic mode meets many of our unmet
interpersonal security needs by providing a means of avoiding anxiety through the clear and mutual interpersonal
expectations of a bureaucratic structure. Diamond's article
describes in detail how the various forms of bureaucracy
create security through obsessional activities, selective
attention and transference. His article serves to underline
the pervasiveness and tenacity of bureaucratic models once
they become entrenched, and provides a caution to dramatic
change in institutional structures without careful attention
to managing the sources of interpersonal stress which will
arise.

The powers of organizational structure also pervade our
cultural base. Denhardt (1981) sees that the organizational
ethic prevails in our everyday lives as an ethic that
emphasizes structure and order over conflict and change. We
could be called the age of structure and organization. The
concern over the impact of bureaucracy on our daily lives is
growing. Hummell (1977) decries our dependency on bureaucracy as a displacement of social norms like love and hate,
freedom and oppression, and justice by the institutional
norms of precision, stability, control and efficiency. We
are in danger of becoming a society without individual
values.

Impact of Bureaucracies on Treatment and Intervention

In human services we are faced with a major crisis. Those
who proclaim that they believe in individualized and
personalized alternatives do so within systems that, by
their very nature, militate against the potential of
individualization. Bureaucratic structures quickly come to
satisfy the security needs of both the staff and disabled
clients at the expense of growth needs of clients.

Some programmes rely on behaviour modification to
ensure acceptable, predictable behaviour. It is a subtle
shift to using behaviour modification to teach compliance
with the attendant reduction of personal control. The
structured interactions of behaviour modification can
isolate staff from meaningful and spontaneous personal
involvement with clients. The current surge in cognitive
behaviour modification and client-managed reinforcement
programmes are, in effect, a recognition of the need to

reverse the dependence on the controls created by earlier forms of behaviour modification.

Individual Programme Planning (IPP) is a powerful tool which facilitates individualization of programmes, but it can result in the opposite effect within entrenched organizational structures. IPPs are easily translated into the *management by objectives* wherein record keeping and accountability overwhelm creative programme planning and client input. IPP systems (and behaviour modification regimes) are popular partly because their consistent structure and ease of mastery appear to provide a way for agencies to use untrained staff rather than hiring trained staff who would encourage creative individual options. IPP use creates the illusion of client involvement. Many IPP systems have been implemented without real commitment to and faith in the ability of disabled people to make their own decisions. Client ideas, even if they are encouraged, are frequently overwhelmed by the weight of professional opinion. In circumstances where clients are involved, their decisions can challenge the neatness of system and cause major problems because clients may not make realistic (i.e. professional) choices.

Wortman (1981) states that ideal voluntary activity as existing in a pre bureaucratic state - in the amorphous edges of societal change in which social movements are formed around configurations of new values. These new values are then translated into service directions. Today, shifting societal values and harsh economic realities mean that flexibility must be maintained at all costs. But it is easy to become resistant to change: inflexibility creeps into large structures and even small established organizations may respond to change in defensive and reluctant ways. Marlett (1978) notes that small group homes may become just as institutionalized and resistant to change as the large facilities for which they were the intended salvation.

Thus we are caught in systems that have powerful seduction in terms of personal, professional and power needs, but that distance us from our purpose. Is it any wonder that professionals have come under attack as neglecting persons with disabilities, becoming disabling professionals (McKnight, 1979; Illich, 1979). But how does one counteract this situation when so much is invested in current structures? First, we need to challenge the dominance of business models and understand the nature of human service organizations. Then, if we choose to aspire to business models we need to seek more relevant business models that will reinforce responsiveness to consumer need.

Challenge to the Corporate Business Model in Rehabilitation

Corporate bureaucracies of business and industry use the manufacturing principles because the success of their business is dependent on a product with consistent quality. The uniformity of the product means the management can be structured in uniform, organized patterns. One can see how technocratic bureaucracies were ideally suited for social welfare models which have as their base universal and equal access to funds. The equity requirement was identical to the uniformity requirement of manufacturing. Hierarchical checks and balances were a reasonable solution. Woodward (1965), in a large British study of manufacturing plants, identifies the role of hierarchical, or bureaucratic management in manufacturing plants, but seriously questions the value of this type of management when customization is required as it is in human services. In rehabilitation, and indeed most human service organizations, we are struggling under the weight of this corporate, manufacturing model - trying to *manufacture* independence by creating a series of *operations* (interventions) through which *raw products* (persons with disability) must pass. Unfortunately, as we can see from Table 1 (adapted from Kouzes and Mico) there is a basic flaw in our reasoning - people will not be content to stay on the assembly line, nor will they conform to our orderly expectations.

TABLE 1   REHABILITATION AND BUSINESS PRINCIPLES

Dimension	Business/Industrial Organizations	Rehabilitation
Manifest motive	Profit and power	Service
Beneficiaries	Owners	Disabled Person
Resource base	Private capital	Public funds
Goals	Unusual and explicit	Individual and diverse
Intervention	Employee-product interactions	Staff-client interaction
Measures of performance	Quantitative	Qualitative

(Adapted from Kouzes & Mico, 1979)

Acceptance of business processes has had to use organizational development approaches to understand and evaluate agencies. While once widely acclaimed within the corporate sectors and public administration, it has very little success or application in the area of small human services (Goldstein, 1978; Weisbord, 1976; Blumberg, 1977; Rubin, Plovnick & Fry, 1977).

Kouzes and Mico (1979) report the problems of organizational development in improving human service organizations, and provide insight into our evolving systems. Domain theory proposes three distinct areas - policy, service and management rather than the single domain assumption of organizational development.

FIGURE 1   GOALS OF THE 3 MAJOR DOMAINS IN HUMAN SERVICE
          ORGANIZATIONS AS OUTLINED IN DOMAIN THEORY

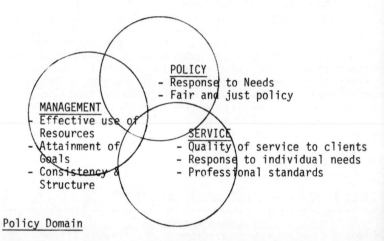

POLICY
- Response to Needs
- Fair and just policy

MANAGEMENT
- Effective use of Resources
- Attainment of Goals
- Consistency & Structure

SERVICE
- Quality of service to clients
- Response to individual needs
- Professional standards

Policy Domain

The policy domain rests with the board of an agency. In the democratic tradition of voluntary associations the membership should approve any of the policy directions or changes proposed by the board. An active consumer membership is the basis of the new independent living models which are emerging and in this they are similar to the parent run organizations of the 50's in their capacity to remain responsive to constituency needs.

In the early stages of evolution of organizations, the policy domain is dominant as needs are identified and means sought to meet the needs. As organizations become more formalized, the policy domain changes both in composition and focus. Whereas initially the board was primarily representative of the consumer, board composition shifts to attract the advisory support needed to run services in the early stages. As boards become more professionalized, the role of the policy domain changes from social action and identifying needs to one of rendering just, impartial and fair policy decisions.

Service Domain

The service domain is usually the next domain to emerge as needs are translated into services. Staff hired by the board share the same commitment to the purposes of the organization and in self help groups some of the staff may come from the board or membership. As the service domain expands, staff grow towards professionalism and want control of their service roles and monitoring quality of service and professional standards. The key to effective service is the ability to respond on an individual basis using a flexible and creative mix of the available processes and methods.

Development of a service domain within rehabilitation has been exciting in Canada and most of the Commonwealth because there were few clearly identified professional rehabilitation training models. Thus professionals in the field of rehabilitation have come from other disciplines, e.g. health, social work, psychology and education. While the development of a coherent service domain has been elusive, it has led to a creative and flexible mix of methodologies within the field. This has meant that the service domain has perhaps had more open boundaries than might otherwise have been the case had we been able to rely on a particular established discipline.

Management Domain

The management domain emerges when the level of service reaches a point where the coordination of resources is no longer conveniently handled by the board or those offering the service. At this point a number of the administrative and funding requirements are transferred to a person or persons who assume the responsibility of bringing order or organizational coherence to the diverse functions within the service domain. Most managers assume that human service organizations should be business-like in their approach, operating on the governing principles of hierarchical control and coordination. Management strives to rationalize the organization, with cost efficiency and effectiveness as the measures of its success.

Domain Interaction

Each domain functions under a separate set of governing principles, measures of success, structural arrangements and work modes. Not only are the characteristics of each domain distinct, they are often incongruent, e.g. management's need for consistency in policy and procedures contrast with the service reality of individual solutions to diverse problems.

In this alone the dilemma of rehabilitation becomes evident. How do we create group treatment procedures for people whose very diversity and complexity is at once both their strength and their greatest need?

Domain theory helps identify the discordance within most human service organizations. While in the business and industrial world, managers are, for the most part, in control of their organizations, managers in human service organizations do not and cannot have the same degree of control. Professionals demand autonomy and self-regulation and the policy domain considers management ultimately accountable to them. Thus it is difficult to achieve coherence within a tri-partite system with management, policy and service each actively vying to maintain stability (Schon, 1971). The existence of multiple domains in human service organizations has led to discordant relationships where different perceptions and contrasting norms prevail, and uncertainty is certain.

Unfortunately, when trying to rationalize systems, we have tended to rely on management based, problem solving techniques - management audits, management by objectives. For the most part these tend to be pragmatic and assume cause effect relationships and common goals. What is required instead is a new breed of managers who understand the discrepancies within the three domains and can recognize and support the various domain values and methods rather than seeking to dominate the system (Kouzes & Mico, 1979).

Facilitators are needed who are able to support the flexibility within a service mode while extracting the consistency and financial order required by government funders. They need to be aware of the very distinct challenges of administrating a tri-partite system wherein they are the liaison - the negotiators rather than the managers. The challenge of management in rehabilitation has never been greater for we are facing increased professionalization of our service domain on one hand, and increased militancy and social action within the consumer/policy domain on the other. We need to strive for harmony, not uniformity within our systems.

In order to move beyond our present stalemate we must address:

1) the irresolvable discrepancies between voluntary human service organizations and business or industrial organizations.
2) the low utility of large corporate structures as the model for rehabilitation.
3) the importance of looking instead at the small service related business as an alternate model for rehabilitation.

Introducing Small Business Methods into Corporate Rehabilitation

While rehabilitation is beginning to embrace technocratic bureaucracy, it is being challenged on its own corporate territory. The current popular business bible, *In Search of Excellence* (Peters & Waterman, 1982), brings to large business and corporate structures the principles of small business management which thrive because of informal and non-hierarchical structures. Peters and Waterman state that effective organizations are built on the smallest unit possible, generate family feelings, focus on simplicity rather than complexity, harness easily identifiable goals and continually reiterate that the human being counts - not only the consumer or the customer but employees as well. Large organizations are realizing that bureaucratic structures or hierarchical structures in many ways prevent responsiveness to change.

Successful private sector executives indicate that they have consciously cut down on corporate systems and staff groupings, streamlined organizations to increase creativity and reduced stifling effects of bureaucracy (Brodtrick & Patton, 1984). Reviews of behaviour of successful managers (Kother, 1982; Mitzberg, 1975) do much to dispel the myth of the cool, organized planful manager we seem to be seeking. Kother found that effective managers work less systematically, more informally, were less organized, less reflective, more reactive and more *frivolous* than their less effective counterparts. In effect they create more responsive, flexible and informal groupings.

In general small business tends to be more creative and innovative because it can afford to learn by making mistakes rather than relying on complex planning processes. In large organizations the cost of risk escalates to the point where agencies become risk averse.

While effectiveness tends to be inversely related to size, i.e. the smaller the group the greater innovation and inventiveness, large organizations can restructure in order to harness the creativity of small informal groups. The Japanese style of management focuses the strengths and creativity of small groups of people within large corporate structures. Small production groups work together to monitor production and to improve their work processes, and companies thereby recognize the importance of individuals within a large corporate structure.

This principle can be applied within most rehabilitation organizations. Day programmes, residential programmes, etc., can be broken down into focus areas - shops, homes, etc., and given autonomy to develop their own unique styles and approaches rather than striving for consistency. Natural and diverse groupings will return to both frontline

87

staff and clients a feeling of control. With control comes motivation, higher performance levels, and more commitment. The ideal solution might be to separate these units and move them throughout the community whereby they can take on the flavour and tone of their neighbourhoods.

This brings us to a second feature in Japanese management - loyalty, commitment, and personal identification with the organization's mission. We need to conscientiously redevelop a *mission* - a unique set of values and goals based on historical characteristics, unique accomplishments or what Burns and Mauet (1984) call *myth-making*. In our desire to become objective and businesslike we have overlooked the basic need to be committed to a purpose. In business, however, mission is essential - a belief in the product and the eventual profit and power which the product will generate. Mission statements form the cognitive maps of the organizations that provide coherent ideologies for daily decision-making (Mitroff & Kilman, 1976). Marlett and Hughson (1979) in their programme evaluation model stress that collective values and beliefs of an organization create a statement of mission that is the essential steering mechanism of a programme blending goals and methods into a functional philosophy; integrating principle (what you say) with practice (what you do). The danger, of course in creating powerful mission statements is that, as organizations decline, these statements will be used by competing organizations as visible examples of standards not met. Nevertheless without mission we are rudderless - operating on policy and routines rather than moving toward coherent goals.

COMMUNITY ECONOMIC DEVELOPMENT - COMMUNITY BASED SMALL BUSINESS

Alternatives

The early sections described the evolution and calcification of rehabilitation as a service industry; this section completes the circle by opening a dialogue of social development for the community of disabled persons. Community economic development is new to the disabled community for a number of reasons:

Economic Impotence:	while there are considerable economic resources allocated to servicing needs of persons with disabilities, they become service rich but money poor.
Clinical Dependence:	one-to-one intervention especially in multidisciplinary terms leaves

	the persons alone, powerless, and often fragmented.
Normalization and Integration:	access to normal life options and equal opportunities has been at the price of rejection of disability as a personal characteristic. Rejection of congregation and deviancy juxtaposition (devalued persons associating or helping each other) often meant that disabled persons were stripped of the natural and meaningful support of mutual help - a secure home base of shared competencies and problems.

All of these factors have left the disabled community behind other disadvantaged groups in asserting their economic self sufficiency.

Economic development does not mean simplistic formulations of self help as the panacea for bureaucratized service although it is founded in a neopopulist perspective that is on the one hand: anti big and anti control from the top, and on the other hand pro community with emphasis on self initiated activities at the grass roots level (Riessman, 1985).

The first section describing the popular conservative process of privatization as a first conceptual attempt at moving services to a community base is followed by the development of professional private practice and consumer managed services as rapidly developing community based alternatives.

Privatization of Long Term Care

There is an upsurge of interest within most conservative governments towards privatization - turning over services traditionally considered to be within the government domain to families and private sector. This is particularly the case in long term residential care. The Province of British Columbia has turned much of their human services over to small independent companies who provide service on a contract basis. After much trial and error, many of these services are responsive to consumer needs. However, the assumption that privatization is the panacea is just as naive as assuming that comprehensive bureaucratic structures are the only way to provide services.

Despite the immense power in privatization to provide responsive service, if we move toward privatization without redressing the current lack of power of disabled persons, we merely transfer ownership of people as commodities from large bureaucracies to small, often hidden, alternatives. Stories of neglect, abuse and frustration are all too common when people, who cannot speak for themselves, are sold to the lowest bidder for servicing. There is also rising concern that governments encourage provision of care by untrained staff because of the costs.

The most direct form of privatization is the provision of financial and programme support to relatives or foster relatives in caring for their disabled family members - in particular children and elderly people. The impact of providing direct family support (financial and personal) on institutionalization can be dramatic. In the 1975/76 Calgary census (Marlett, 1984) only 12 per cent of medically dependent youngsters under five were in their own home or community alternative. There was a dramatic change in the 1977/78 census to 86 per cent living at home. The development of infant intervention, family support, respite care and primarily government financial assistance made it possible for families to help their children at home. Further, the age at admission to institutions in 1970 to 1974 was 2.9 years, but by 1978 to 1982 the average age at admission had risen to just over 10 years.

While financial assistance to families has reduced use of public institutions it can cause severe hardship for relatives unless sensitive personal support is provided. Mellor et al. (1982), in a powerful report on partnership for change called *A Blue Print for Social Action*, provide a model that all of us in the field of rehabilitation should study in developing small home based alternatives to institutional care for persons requiring extensive personal care. They discuss the positive impact of providing individual services to families caring for frail and older relatives. They also indicate that the main stress factor in such arrangements is the loss of self identity of the care giver. In devoting time and energy to a frail older person the care giver loses perspective of his or her own self, and invests much of their identity in someone else's life. This can lead to anger and frustration, guilt and a increasing lack of self-worth and fear of abuse.

Luckily Mellor's programme provided opportunities for care givers to get together on a regular basis and thereby allowed the natural support of a self-help group to emerge among care givers. The support staff to the care givers, were aware of the dangers inherent in staff co-opting the group process. They supported the needs of the care givers' autonomy but provided a forum for education and group action and this, in turn, fostered individual feelings of worth and support. Both a care givers' network and a professional coalition have emerged. These do not seek to join forces, but collaborate when needed.

Community home care for physically disabled adults, another option for privatized long term solutions, has opened many doors to a more natural and fulfilling life, and few would argue that it is economically advantageous for persons to live in their own home with supports provided as needed. However planning home care services must be done with and by consumers to avoid feelings of helplessness, loneliness and constant fear of neglect. At the present time we have two ends of a continuum for the provision of home care support:

1) independent, where the individual is responsible for recruiting training, monitoring and paying the attendant and

2) institutional, where home care monopolies (often government sponsored) provide comprehensive services including a single entry, coordinated service contact by agency staff with mandated financial guidelines and programmes.

If the individual opts for independent management, he or she may be faced with total responsibility and few safety nets. Living under constant threat of attendants not showing up and the constant worry of finding replacements can lead the most fiercely independent person to retreat to a custodial setting. On the other hand, the current trend toward institutionalization of community care leaves the disabled person at the mercy of a bureaucratized administration. Professional support staff and attendants travelling between clients are often severely limited in the time allotted for each person and the type of care they can give. Group prescriptions (medications, technical aides, nursing supplies) rob the disabled person of personal choice, neighbourhood support and creative solutions. Obviously there must be a compromise - one which maximizes the opportunities for individual solutions while providing security for attendants and a safety net for the independent disabled person.

There is a further concern that privatizing services for disadvantaged persons is becoming a convenient yet covert method for political patronage.

Professional Private Practice

The move toward small business alternatives from large professional bureaucracies is reflected in the growing number of professionals entering *private practice*. In allied health areas such as physiotherapy and speech therapy, specialized clinics are being established outside of hospital with medical referral providing access to health care dollars. Counselling clinics, psychological services and remedial education services have also become a common practice within some communities (in some entire fee is paid by the consumer, in others, health care insurance covers the cost). In rehabilitation there is a wide variety of individuals who feel that they have services to offer disabled consumers, and are willing to work on a fee for service basis, especially if the disabled consumers have purchasing power. It takes courage and financial resources to move outside of secure bureaucratic structure into the uncertainties of a hand to mouth existence. Some large organizations and government structures provide support during the establishment phase of small companies seeing the generation of alternatives as a healthy sign rather than a thrust. Professional training programmes are beginning to train free lance professionals to be able to move creatively in the community. To do this, the new professional must be challenged to think independently, to analyze situations and to form alliances with often unlikely business partners. If small independent alternatives are going to survive we must learn how to work together through networks i.e. sharing information and referrals and providing needed support to each other. Employee benefits, such as medical plans and insurance, and small business supports such as accounting, space and equipment, and receptionists, can also be shared in creative cooperative alliances thereby lessening the emotional and financial overhead of operating independently.

Consumer Managed Services

The processes of community economic development wherein a community - be it geographic or cultural - provides its own services is well established within ethnic groups, women and disadvantaged districts, but the disabled community is only now moving to develop and offer services to its constituents. The independent living centres in the United States have pioneered community economic development offering housing, transportation, technical aid, attendant care, vacation assistance, etc. These services tend to remain small and responsive because they offer direct and personalized service to a target group who have not only a vested interest but representation on management boards. That is not to say that they will not face the same subtle seduction to grow into bureaucratic structures but the direct and personal nature of the service makes depersonalization more difficult.

Infrastructures for Social Development

Small business can provide exciting alternatives to institution services, but society must always be aware of the motives in turning care over to the private sector lest in the process we open doors to reduction in the level of support while removing from public attention the need for accountability and responsibility of government (Marino, 1984).

Small service providers, while responsive and flexible, face arbitrary hurdles in establishing government support for funding because most government funders prefer to fund large bureaucratic services. For example, in the Province of Alberta agencies have to agree to serve a minimum of 50 persons before being considered for vocational rehabilitation grants. This prevents the development of innovative solutions in favour of established processes because of the risk factors - it is difficult to start new alternatives on a large scale! Despite the obstacles small business service alternatives have emerged in many areas - group homes, career placement, family support and behavioural consultation. Consumer and staff satisfaction appears high in these options, but funding will likely continue to be a problem until basic approaches to evaluation and accountability within these small models are brought more into line with their functions.

Governments are trying to ensure accountability by stipulating that small business services must be operated by non-profit societies who can be held accountable for the level of care provided to persons in their facilities as if the continuance of the charity ethic ensured dedication to quality. This mix of small business and voluntary organization models can lead to strange combinations - entrepreneurs who must find token boards to meet regulations or non profit groups (e.g. churches, parent groups, consumer co-ops) trying to operate small businesses without small business knowledge.

Self Help Clearing Houses in the United States and Canada provide support to existing and emerging self-help groups (e.g. California Self-Help Clearing Houses, Montreal) in an innovative support network. They provide resource information for self-help groups, assistance in recruiting members, support in social action processes, community organization, and public education.

If disabled persons are going to be able to take advantage of community based services the following issues must be addressed:

1) transfer of financial power from agency based funding to the person with the disability, i.e. the consumer.

2) mechanisms which facilitate the access to and coordination of needed supports.

3) means of building personal support networks that will prevent people becoming *lost in society*.

The independent living movement attempts to provide the impetus for these three factors. Consumer controlled centres mobilize the power mutual aid (peer support) and social action (advocacy) within a community development framework.

1. Funding the Individual

Success of the Independent Living Model rests on establishing personal financial control over services and supports. Considerable purchasing power would be available if one combined the subsidy allowances, the per diem programme costs and professional fees into one sum. This then could be allocated to the disabled individual or a volunteer committee who would coordinate and manage service requirements. The independent living allocations in the United States promote disabled persons becoming managers of their own services. In this, the option exists for disabled individuals to pool their existing subsidies and reserves, to set up independent accommodation and purchase the services they require. British Columbia, Alberta and Ontario are also experimenting with the concept of funding following the individual, although this is being done primarily through the home care allocations for attendant care. The current focus is on physically disabled and elderly persons, but the same principles apply to mentally disabled persons who require supportive personal guidance instead of personal care assistance.

The accountability of privatization increases dramatically when purchasing power is vested with the disabled individual, his family or advocacy committees. In the ideal situation of service alternatives and a buyers' market, operators would be faced with the necessity of providing quality service or the individual would go elsewhere. The threat of competition would increase accountability and the level of responsiveness. Unfortunately we are faced with a seller's market in the service field with more buyers than services available.

2. Mechanisms to Facilitate Access to and Coordination of Services

An essential difference between professional and social development models rests in the access to information. When professionals control information, the person with the disability is always dependent. Free and full access to information is a keystone of the Canadian approach to independent living. Centres become a community nexus of information related to disability and services - providing a peer support back up when individuals require assistance in using or understanding the information. Service registries, (housing, attendant care) and assistance in managing services provide the backup system for those living independently.

Service brokerage provides financial services which support individual solutions. It involves acting with or on behalf of others in negotiating ongoing service agreements which facilitate consumer control and independent living. Brokerage empowers the consumer through vesting purchasing power and accountability with the individual. It encourages self advocacy and peer support in negotiating with existing and developing systems and developing resources. It requires training and safety nets for individuals who are managing their services independently.

While still in its infancy, this concept perhaps holds one solution to providing individualized and consumer managed services for individuals who lack the experience/-confidence or the ability to be totally independent. Brokerage is fraught with dangers of amalgamating business practice and human service. The major concern in the establishment of brokerage systems is maintaining brokers who are indeed free of a conflict of interest. Service providers should not become service brokers nor should service brokers evolve into providing services lest the independence of advocacy be compromised. This is extraordinarily difficult when service provision is still not responsive to individual needs.

3. Means of Building Personal Support

Peer support and counselling can provide support and assistance for those individuals who are moving toward independent management of their resources. Those who have been through similar processes can provide information and referral services, assist in managing services, and in general, provide the safety net as individuals move from highly supportive and structured environments into often unresponsive community environments. In the initial stages of transition from professionally run services to consumer purchased services such intermediate supports are essential. Without them we negate the rights of a large percentage of persons who are not, at the present time, capable of managing all of their resources.

For those persons for whom informal supports are not sufficient, a more formal personal support network may be needed. The Joshua Committee (*for when the walls came tumbling down*) was formed around Judy Snow by seven close associates to provide a functional in-home personal care system. It is a good example of the potential power of people working together to advocate for more personalized and consumer controlled services. Joshua Committees or circles also have potential when looking at the needs of those who may need support and guidance in making realistic decisions for themselves. The Community Living Committee of Vancouver, a group of interested parents, maximize personalized life choices for individuals by advocating and purchasing services on their behalf. This could also happen when a committee of friends of disabled persons agree to become the trustee of the funds, working with the individual to build a support system of creative alternatives. In one such example an independent service broker from the Calgary Association of Independent Living, along with an informal network of friends, have built a caring and creative independent living alternative for a young brain injured man who had been refused services by all community services because of his behaviour. In a personalized environment where he has meaningful control and respect he has learned to be a roommate, a friend, an explorer and most important, his own personal advocate.

The real strength of the independent living movement rests in the as yet untapped capacity of people to care about each other. Persons with disabilities can and do support each other, but more importantly, the independent living movement is not an exclusive club - any one can belong, even professionals.

SUMMARY

This chapter has attempted to deal from a number of perspectives with the institutionalization of rehabilitation services. It has tried to provide some conceptual models for understanding both existing services and alternatives which exist outside of the traditional rehabilitation structures. Finally it has tried to provide a number of alternatives to our traditional concept of rehabilitation services.

A number of major concepts have been introduced:

1) the importance of theories and models in organizing our behaviour,
2) the role of service delivery models in rehabilitation
    - welfare
    - professional
    - self help
    - social action
    - partnership,

3) the theory and impact of technocratic bureaucracies on rehabilitation,
4) how services and interventions become changed because of business models and the nature of human service organizations as distinct from technocratic bureaucracies,
5) policy, service and management domains,
6) challenge to the corporate business model,
7) community economic development and small business principles as evident in privatization, private practice and independent living centres,
8) social development infrastructure such as funding for individuals, brokerage, personal support networks.

REFERENCES

Bandler, R., & Grinder, J. (1975) *The Structure of Magic*, (Vol.1), Science & Behavior Books, Palo Alto, California.

Blumberg, A. (1977) 'A Complex Problem - An Overly Simple Diagnosis, *Journal of Applied Behavioral Science, 13*(2), 184-189.

Brodtrick, O. & Patton, R. (1984) 'Managing Within the Public Sector,' *Supply and Services, Canada Bureau of Manpower, 15*(1).

Brown, R. I. (1984) *Integrated Programmes for Handicapped Adolescents and Adults*, Croom Helm, Beckenham, U.K.

Burns, M. & Mauet, A. (1984) 'Administrative Freedom for Interorganizational Action - A Life Cycle Interpretation,' *Administration and Society, 16*(3), 289-305.

Denhardt, R. B. (1981) *In the Shadow of Organization*, The Regence Press of Kansas, Lawrence.

Diamond, M. A. (1984) 'Bureaucracy as Externalized Self Esteem,' *Administration and Society, 16*(2), August, 195-214

Goldstein, L. D. (1978) *Consulting with Human Service Systems*, Addison-Wesley, Reading, Massachusetts.

Heller, T. & Van Til, J. (1983) 'Changing Authority Patterns and the Future of Institutional Management,' in M. S. Moyer (ed.), *Managing Voluntary Organizations*, Faculty of Administrative Studies, York University.

Hummell, R. (1977) *The Bureaucratic Experience*, St. Martin's Press, New York.

Illich, I. (1979) *Disabling Professions*, Harper and Row, New York.

Kother, M. (1982) 'What Effective Managers Really Do,' *Harvard Business Review, 60*(6), 156-167.

Kouzes, J. M., & Mico, P. R. (1979) 'Domain Theory: An Introduction to Organizational Behavior in Human Service Organizations,' *The Journal of Applied Behavioral Science, 15,* 449-469.

Kuhn, T. (1962) *Structure of Scientific Revolutions,* University of Chicago Press, Chicago.

Marino, R. (1984) 'Self Help - A Complement to the Welfare State or a Neo-Conservative Ploy?' Paper for 25th Annual Conference of the Western Association of Sociology and Anthropology, Regina, Saskatoon.

Marlett, N. J. (1978) 'Normalization, Socialization and Integration,' in J. P. Das, & D. Baine (eds.), *Mental Retardation for Special Educators,* C. C. Thomas, Springfield, Illinois.

Marlett, N. J. (ed.) (1984) *Disability Information System of Calgary 1983 Census,* Community HORIZONS '84, Calgary.

Marlett, N. J. & Hughson, E. A. (1979) *Rehabilitation Programs Manual,* Vocational and Rehabilitation Research Institute, Calgary.

McKnight, J. (1979) 'Professionalized Service and Disabling Help,' in I. Illich, *Disabling Professions,* Harper and Row, New York.

Mellor, J., et al. (1982) 'Partnership of Caring: A Blueprint for Social Action,' ERDS document publication.

Mitroff, I. & Kilman, R. (1976) 'On Organizational Stories: An Approach to the Design and Analysis of Organizations Through Myths and Stories,' in R. Kilman, *The Management of Organizational Design, Vol. 1, Strategies and Implementation,* North Holland, New York.

Mitzberg, A. (1975) 'The Manager's Job: Folklore and Fact,' *Harvard Business Review, 53*(4), 49-61.

Peters, T. J. & Waterman, Jr. R. H. (1982) *In Search of Excellence: Lessons from America's Best-Run Companies,* Harper and Row, New York.

Riessman, F. (1985) 'New Dimensions in Self Help,' *Social Policy, Winter,* 2-4.

Rubin, I., Plovnick, M., & Fry, R. (1977) 'The Role of the Consultant in Initiating Planned Change: A Case Study in Health Care Systems,' in W. W. Burke (ed.), *Current Issues and Strategies in Organization Development,* Human Sciences Press, New York.

Salamon, L. (1983) 'Non Profit Organizations and the Rise of Third Party Government: The Scope, Character and Consequences of Government Support of Non Profit Organization in Independent Sector,' in M. S. Moyer (ed.), *Managing Voluntary Organizations,* Conference proceedings published by Faculty of Administrative Studies, York University.

Schon, D. A. (1971) *Beyond the Stable State,* Norton, New York.

Trist, E. (1977) 'Collaboration in Work Settings: A Personal Perspective,' *Journal of Applied Behavioral Science, 13* (3), 268-278.

Weber, M. (1948) 'Max Weber Essays in Sociologies,' in H. H. Gerth, & C. W. Mills, (eds.), *Sociology,* Oxford University Press, London.

Weber, M. (1968) 'On Charisma and Institution Building' in S. W. Eisenhadt (ed.), University of Chicago Press, Chicago.

Weisbord, M. P. (1976) 'Why Organization Development Hasn't Worked (So Far) in Medical Centers,' *Health Care Management Review, 1* (Spring), 17-28.

Woodward, J. (1965) *Industrial Organization: Theory and Practice,* Oxford University Press, London.

Wortman, Jr., M. S. (1981) 'A Radical Shift from Bureaucracy to Strategic Management in Voluntary Organizations,' *Journal of Voluntary Action Research, 10,* 62-81.

Chapter Six

CONJOINT EVALUATION AS A PROGRAMME DEVELOPMENT STRATEGY

Ralph Westwood

INTRODUCTION: WHY EVALUATE

Historical Overview

Since the history of the North American movement to assess and treat persons with disabilities dates back to the beginning of this century, one could assume that there should be a history that affects both our understanding of the process and our need to know how well the process is working. One way to conceptualize this development is to consider the varying answers that have been given over the years to the question: why should we evaluate? If we look at this issue in three fairly distinct time periods, beginning in 1910, we find that the answers have changed dramatically with each shift in the way society viewed its persons with disabilities (Frey, 1984):

1. To care for those who are less fortunate (1910-1940). The purpose of evaluation was to determine whether the programme met the basic needs of its clients in a cost effective manner.
2. To rehabilitate people with impairments (1940-1960). Evaluation was directed to determine how effectively programmes and services assisted persons with disabilities in using their existing capacities to develop as fully as possible.
3. To prepare persons with disabilities for life in the mainstream of society (since 1960). Evaluation stresses service accountability and responsiveness to the needs of the individuals. It also accentuates multidisciplinary services and programmes monitoring the quality of these services. In many instances, the requirements are reflected in guidelines, accreditation standards, or legislation affecting the service (DeJong & Lifchez, 1983).

100

The shifts in focus occurred in a cumulative fashion, rather than each replacing the previous concern. It is also important to note that evaluation of rehabilitation programmes is occurring in an increasingly complex system. This point is made not to stress the possible confusion that can occur, but to indicate that practitioners must be prepared to work within a system that is becoming more sophisticated. The answer to *why evaluate* now is: to improve the programme's efficiency, effectiveness, and environmental impact (Schalock, 1983).

This chapter addresses a number of issues specific to the implementation and evaluation of new rehabilitation and special education programmes. Because these programmes are unique to the extent that they are established and funded to meet the needs of people with specific disabilities, they frequently require special information sharing mechanisms to develop effectively and to maintain the support of the interest groups concerned with the services they provide. Before expanding upon some of the characteristics of programmes for persons with disabilities, the concerns of specific interest groups, and the strengths of conjoint evaluation, two frequently used terms must be defined.

Conjoint programme evaluation is a method of evaluation where the programme operator and the agency funding the programme work in combination, over an extended period of time, to design an evaluation plan, collect and analyse data, and summarize findings, in order to understand what the programme does, and how well it achieves its purpose and objectives.

Evaluation is a set of procedures designed to obtain information about the functioning of a programme and to appraise programme merit.

In order to understand how conjoint evaluation can be an effective programme evaluation approach, a brief review of some of the features of programmes for persons with disabilities may be useful.

1. Many persons with disabilities have individual needs that require affirmative and special programmes to reduce some of the disadvantages of the disability. In addition, because these people comprise only a small portion of the public, their needs are often brought to the attention of funding agencies and the public by politically active special interest groups composed of parents, persons with disabilities, and other concerned individuals.

2. Because the level of public involvement with programmes for persons with disabilities is generally quite limited, ongoing assurances of support can be quite capricious especially if the programme is competing with other worthy causes for resources.

3. The purposes and objectives of special programmes have not been widely understood. Often, they were established *to do something* because regular programmes were deemed inappropriate or unavailable. Recent changes in training technology and legislation have resulted in new expectations and the pursuit of concepts such as: normalization, least restrictive alternative, competitive employment, independence, and quality of life (Beasley, 1984). It is worth noting that the various concerned groups have not reached consensus on what constitutes adequate and appropriate services.

4. Special programmes, because of their intensity and range of services, tend to be significantly more expensive than programmes provided for non-disabled persons. They are rarely financed by user fees and must rely on funding from public revenues, corporations, and service agencies. This special funding requirement is the basis of the relationship of shared programme responsibility that exists between the programme operators and the agencies that provide funding (Elliott, 1980; Topliss, 1982).

5. Often, new programmes for persons with disabilities begin as demonstration or pilot programmes with limited statements of purpose. One of the primary objectives usually centres on clearly defining what kind of service is required. Often, however, there is no mechanism in place after the programme begins that assists both parties to reach a shared understanding of the programme's activities and future goals. Divergence or disagreement on programme purpose will tend to jeopardize further programme development.

6. In the past evaluations done to request or support continuing funding, were frequently quite superficial and subjective. Many were solely prepared by the programme operator, while the funding agency and other concerned groups remained unaware of how the data was obtained. As a result, these parties frequently had incomplete and conflicting perceptions of the effectiveness of the programme.

With this history, it is not surprising that programme operators and funding agencies have recently shown greater interest in evaluation. They are looking for processes that will provide the kind of information needed to understand mutually the strengths and weaknesses of programmes. At the same time, it is required that the process reinforce responsibility and accountability.

This chapter reviews developmental stages of new programmes, expectations of various special interest groups, and nine major components of conjoint evaluation, and concludes with general observations about:

- the increasing interest in the accountability of human service programmes,
- the effectiveness of conjoint evaluation, and
- suggested information collection techniques.

COMMON APPROACHES TO EVALUATION

Ideally, if an evaluation procedure is well designed, any changes in student/client skills, or other results attributable to the programme should be measurable. This kind of evaluation normally requires a level of control over the environment that is not feasible or ethical in developing educational and human service programmes. Indeed the purpose of programme evaluation referred to in this chapter is not to add to the body of scientific knowledge, but to obtain reasonably accurate information about the use of specific techniques and the functions and products of a programme. This can be gathered by much less stringent methods.

Evaluators are often concerned about the need to reconcile the apparent conflict between *subjective* judgments and *objective* science. In human service programmes, they should be careful not to get *bogged down* in controversies about the evaluation processes. It is much more productive to first determine the purpose of the programme and then select the best available methods to determine whether the programme is achieving it (Fink & Kosecoff, 1984).

Evaluation is often divided into two broad categories: formative and summative evaluation. Both categories require that several common steps be taken:

1. Identify the programme purpose and objectives.
2. Determine if the purpose and objectives have changed since the programme began. If so how and why?
3. Identify performance standards relevant to the programme objectives.
4. Try to identify some of the unanticipated consequences of the programme.
5. Adopt or develop appropriate methods of measuring important programme outcome.
6. Adopt or develop techniques to determine whether specific programme outcome resulted from the activities of the programme or was due to other causes.
7. Reach agreement with the various concerned groups on both the evaluation format and process to be used.
8. Identify the costs and likely benefits of the evaluation process (Schalock, 1983).

The formative and summative approaches to evaluation differ most in relation to purpose and timing. For example, formative evaluation is an ongoing process designed to gather information for the purpose of taking timely action in order to revise and improve the quality of a programme (Schmuck et al., 1977). It is based on a principle of professionalism where the programme staff are seen to be competent and highly motivated to work toward refinement of their programme. It also assumes an administrative environment in which the programme is highly accountable to its students/clients for the services provided. Essentially, formative evaluation in the context that it is used here is part of a feedback process, where data is collected about the activities of the programme and the effect that those activities have on the students/clients.

Formative evaluation requires that data be collected at frequent intervals or on a continuous basis and that they be regularly analyzed. Decisions reached as a result are based on experience. Formative evaluation allows teachers, instructors, therapists, and others to serve better their students/clients by systematically collecting programme data that will help diagnose areas of strength and weakness. Formative evaluation is designed to answer the following kinds of questions (Flynn & Boschen, 1984):

- Did specific goals or objectives actually get implemented as planned?
- What actually happened in accomplishing a particular task?
- What approach or approaches work better than others?
- How and why were particular procedures modified?
- What can be done to modify a particular approach so that it will work better?

Summative evaluation is the compilation of information about a project or a programme for the purpose of reaching a value judgement about it (Schmuck et al., 1977). Summative evaluation is designed to answer questions like:

- What was the overall effectiveness of the programme?
- Did the programme achieve its purpose?
- Was the programme implemented as designed?
- What components of the programme were most effective?
- What initial goals were achieved that can be used as a baseline for a future evaluation?

Several important issues need to be addressed before preparing to carry out either of these evaluations. The answers to the following questions should be known and agreed upon by the various special interest groups involved well before the process is initiated:

- What are the major questions to be answered by the evaluation?
- What programme areas should be addressed?
- What will be the important indicators of success?
- Can the required data be collected?
- What are the time and resource limitations?
- How will the evaluation results be reported and used?

Development of the evaluation format should involve all of the directly affected special interest groups. It is important to decide what will be reviewed, what the performance indicators will be, who will be responsible for doing the evaluation, and how the results will be reported. These are issues that affect many people. The concerned groups or their representatives should be informed and consulted about the evaluation in advance.

STAGES IN PROGRAMME DEVELOPMENT AND EXPECTATIONS OF THE PROGRAMME

When a decision is made to evaluate a new programme, there are a number of variables to be considered with regard to the effect that they can have on the evaluation process and the final results. Two variables that often cause evaluators considerable concern are:

- maturation of the programme as it is being evaluated, and
- the challenge of attempting to integrate the numerous expectations of special interest groups.

Often evaluation results are questioned because they do not account for the rapid changes that occur in new programmes, or the evaluation did not adequately consider expectations of various concerned interest groups.

As new programmes are created and grow, they move through five quite distinct stages:

1) initiation,
2) start-up,
3) situational analysis,
4) design and implementation, and
5) formal evaluation and adjustment.

Concern about evaluation is usually focused on the final stage; however, the importance of monitoring essential programme development and fine-tuning activities should also be addressed at each of the earlier stages (Johnston et al., 1978).

The following discussion on stages of programme development is geared to conjoint programme development, where both the programme operator and the funding agency are in accord on the programme purpose.

Stage 1: Initiation

The programme operator and the funding agency must agree at this point that there is a need to be met and that they will work together to address it. Before this stage is reached a parent group, an association for disabled persons, or a government agency may have worked for many months or years to document the need, publicize the issue and find agencies willing to provide the required service and funding (Beasley, 1984).

Stage 2: Start-up

At this stage, the programme will often be considered a pilot or demonstration project and the agreement between the programme operator and the funding agency should specify: a) service need, b) what is to be done, c) when and where the programme will be provided, d) how the programme will be organized, and e) any constraints or conditions under which the programme must operate, such as criterion for student/client eligibility, duration of the programme, funding level, and time until a formal evaluation will be completed.

Stage 3: Situational Analysis

Although every programme is unique with regard to purpose, environment, resources, and many other major variables, the diagnostic process is usually quite similar. It normally begins by confirming the service demand, describing existing services, identifying required services, defining tasks and roles to be performed, determining which skills and personnel are required, and identifying delivery problems. This diagnosis also involves how the work should be organized, coordinated and rewarded. The initial evaluation questions and feedback mechanisms are often relatively easy to plan at this stage.

Stage 4: Design and Implementation

This stage normally occurs over a period of several months and involves a number of linkages as a *system* is put into place. The objectives, standards, tasks, jobs, and expected results need to be defined. Developing the evaluation plan well before the programme is implemented enforces a deliberate, careful and systematic approach to actual implementation. It is very important at this stage to build in check points indicating how the programme will reach the various milestones in its development. Implementation may proceed slowly with the orientation and training of new personnel, but it is often characterized by considerable excitement about creating something new. This is normally tempered with the realization that since it is new, care must be taken to ensure that it is *on target* and that a series of initial goals are achieved within the first few months. The writer was recently involved with a vocational training programme that felt compelled to expand its services before satisfying itself that the initial goals were properly reached. Soon it was evident they could no longer cope as the pressures of new and varied responsibilities started to assert themselves. It was finally necessary to cut back services and reinitiate the start-up stages again.

Stage 5: Formal Evaluation and Adjustment

At the end of a predetermined period the evaluation data are collected, analyzed, and the results formally summarized to determine programme success. This period of *stock taking* occurs in addition to continuous programme monitoring, which is required to make ongoing programme changes.

Adjustment refers to the introduction of new information into the development process by repeating portions of stage 3 (situation analysis) and stage 4 (design and implementation). This provides an opportunity to make any necessary changes, before re-evaluating.

SPECIAL PROBLEMS FOR PROGRAMME ADJUSTMENT

The organizational and social environments of programmes change as they mature, and this has important implications for evaluation. A new programme, or a change in an existing programme, presents a great opportunity to create a sharply focused social and technological environment that can be effective in addressing a particular service need. However, start-up situations can pose at least two special problems for programme evaluation.

First, there are often no useful pre-programme measures. Those measures that may be available for a redeveloped programme are likely to be irrelevant. For these reasons, the classic *before and after* comparisons are not normally possible.

107

Second, environmental conditions similar to the *Hawthorne Effect* frequently exist in a new programme. The people and the programme can be dramatically affected by all of the excitement and attention that can occur at start-up. This strong positive response can, if not viewed within the proper context, be misinterpreted in the evaluation results. Figure 1 shows that, beginning with launch and development, programmes go through three distinct stages of maturation, each stage presents a different environmental situation for the programme and its personnel (Johnston et al., 1978).

FIGURE 1 STAGES OF PROGRAMME MATURATION

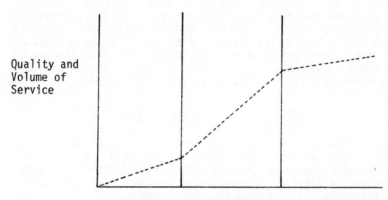

Quality and
Volume of
Service

Launch and   Stabilization
Development   and Refinement Mature Operation

During launch and development, people are primarily engaged in orientation, preparation and piloting. The tasks are still likely to be fragmented and people may not yet be working together on the ultimate purpose of the programme. Some may bide their time to see how the programme develops, while others will assume that the programme will continue much as it is at this stage. For these reasons, general observations should only be tentative, given the short-term and artificial nature of the situation.

In the stabilization and refinement stage, the atmosphere is often highly charged with excitement by the dual pressures of providing a necessary service and refining the service delivery vehicle. The situation can be very satisfying to people motivated by the challenge and the evidence of activity; it can also be threatening to those who are uncomfortable with change. Some people are highly motivated by the dynamic conditions that can exist during this stage and they respond very positively when asked their opinion. Later, when things slow down and programme activities are more routine, they may feel much less positive and involved.

It is well known in the construction industry that some people are *start-up gypsies*, they travel from one site to another seeking the adventure of the launch and stabiliz- ation stages, but then move on again when the programme matures (Johnston et al., 1978). This phenomenon can also affect persons and interest groups not directly involved. They too may be overly impressed by the promise and activity of a new programme as it begins. Collecting personal perception data at this stage can be misleading without an awareness of this phenomenon.

Most of the initial corrective actions have already occurred by onset of the mature operation stage. The work environment has established itself and the relationships among people and with organizations in the system should also be settled. It is only during this third stage that one can speak of *normal* programme activities. The programme ceases to be so concerned about its own creation, and is much more focused on its product, relationships with others, long range purposes, level of service, and standards. More conclusive evaluation results of overall programme effectiveness are possible; however, it may take three years or more to reach this stage. This feature of programme development and maturation must be carefully considered when evaluation results are used to determine future programme funding. If the purpose of evaluation is to measure programme need or its effectiveness, it is obvious that the programme should be allowed to mature beyond the launch and stabilization stages before the evaluation is completed.

THE ORIENTATION AND EXPECTATIONS OF SPECIAL INTEREST GROUPS

Special interest groups have strong expectations. They often view programmes as vehicles to resolve or address needs that they have identified. The degree to which a particular programme is successful depends upon how well its purpose addresses the various needs and how effectively it is implemented. The programmes discussed are:

1) educational and service programmes, designed to serve people with disabilities, and
2) programmes that train specialists to provide services required by persons with disabilities.

There are usually five separate special interest groups directly or indirectly concerned with the programme:

1) students/clients have unfulfilled needs and require a service;
2) programme operators wish to provide a service and request financial assistance to do so;
3) funding agencies agree that a service should be provided and they are willing, subject to certain conditions, to support a programme operator in doing so;
4) lobby groups represent the interests and special needs of students/clients and recommend that certain services should be provided; and
5) other interest groups represent the interests of funding agencies, taxpayers, stockholders, or other organizations.

When a programme is being developed, at least the programme operator and funding agency agree to work together to achieve a common purpose. Although they share responsibility for the programme, they come to the situation from different perspectives. They have varying sets of expectations; some are commonly held and others are not (Townsend, 1981). While it is useful for all special interest groups to be aware of the expectations of the others, it is particularly important for the programme operator and the funding agency to understand each other. All special interest groups have at least one common expectation: that the service provided will be a benefit to the student/client. Some of the expectations commonly held by each special interest group (for example, Accreditation Council for Facilities for the Mentally Retarded, 1980; Alberta Education, 1985) are:

Students/Clients - That the service be delivered in a convenient and helpful fashion and that it be sensitive to individual needs.
- That the service provider be interested in the student's/client's perceptions of the service, and not change or discontinue the service without consultation.

Programme Operator- That the funding agency provide adequate funding to allow the programme to achieve its purpose.
- That the programme continue as long as there is a need for its service.
- That the student/client and the other special interest groups understand what the programme is trying to accomplish and appreciate the service provided.

Funding Agency   - That the programme be operated in an efficient and effective manner.
                      - That the programme operator regularly communicate with the funding agency about the general functioning of the programme.
                      - That the results achieved by the programme reflect positively on the funding agency.

Lobby Groups   - That they be consulted about the achievements of the programme and any changes planned.
                      - That the service be improved and updated whenever possible.
                      - That their advice and counsel be sought and seriously considered.

Other Interested   - That the service not compete with or
Parties   reduce grouped parties' resources available to other programmes.
                      - That the programme be operated as effectively and efficiently as possible.
                      - That they be informed from time-to-time on the general purpose and results of the service.

With this range of expectations in mind, it is obvious that there should be a mechanism in place to ensure that the programme operator, funding agency, and the other interested groups are kept well informed about the effectiveness of the programme. Some general approaches are good community and public relations, publicizing programme activities, and encouraging personal contact with the programme. Conjoint programme evaluation is a specific mechanism that can strengthen the link between the programme operator and the funding agency.

It is not uncommon to find human service programmes that start out in a near adversarial relationship with their funding agency and other concerned individuals, especially following a long campaign to obtain funding. This can be the basis of future problems unless the programme operator and funding agency reach agreement about their expectations for the programme. It is essential that this issue is resolved and put aside so that future energies can be focused on improving the quality of student/client services. Programme evaluation should not be seen as just a tool of the funding agency, programme administration or legislative body; rather it can be a tool for constructive planning and service improvement (Kiernan & Petzy, 1982).

111

WHAT ARE THE COMPONENTS OF AN EFFECTIVE CONJOINT EVALUATION DESIGN?

A conjoint evaluation design is most feasibly developed following a review of the purpose of the evaluation and the circumstances that are specific to the programme. Since conjoint evaluation involves both a process of data gathering to learn about the programme and *stock-taking* to reach conclusions on its merit, the reader will notice that conjoint evaluation uses elements of both formative and summative evaluation. The nine basic steps in conjoint evaluation design are:

1. <u>Agree to conjointly evaluate</u>. An agreement is required between the programme operator and the funding agency on how they will work together cooperatively to satisfy their mutual needs for information about the programme. Their respective needs for information can best be met through conjoint development of an evaluation design that gives direction to the evaluation process. Participation by programme personnel and other persons who can assist in the design process can be extremely useful. Their role should be to assist in confirming the programme purpose, objectives, and standards that should be considered by the evaluation.

2. <u>Agree on the purpose, objectives and standards of the programme</u>. If a programme was initially well planned, its purpose and objectives will reflect the student/-client needs identified by concerned individuals, associations, literature, experts, and programme planners. If the programme purpose and objectives were never formally stated, it must be done at this stage because a programme cannot be evaluated without knowing what it is supposed to do. Having to clarify the objectives at this late stage is unfortunate because it tends to narrow the focus of the evaluation to current programme objectives, rather than to the informal objectives that existed when the programme was implemented (Fink & Kosecoff, 1984). In either case, the first step in the evaluation design is to confirm the purpose and objectives, and to identify which of the objectives should be included in the evaluation process.
    When a number of objectives have been initially agreed upon, each should be linked to a specific standard so that it is possible to determine when the objective has been achieved. For example, a major objective of transition programmes is to prepare graduates for employment. A number of questions about standards quickly come to mind.

- Does employment mean competitive, sheltered, or other?
- Is part-time employment sufficient?
- What is part-time?
- Is there a basic wage requirement?
- Will unrelated employment be included in this objective?

Acceptable standards may be derived from professional practice, accreditation bodies, experience gained from similar programmes, or information from the current literature (Commission on Accreditation of Rehabilitation Facilities, 1984). For example, a planning group concerned with teaching reading skills to adults with hearing impairments will need to struggle with the content and age appropriateness of the various standards. Existing standards may need to be significantly modified and the group must also determine whether certain objectives are measurable and, therefore, useful for judging programme success (Kiernan & Petzy, 1984). Selecting the objectives and standards should be a logical process, and care should be taken to avoid making it unnecessarily complex.

3. Identify what each of the special interest groups needs to know over short-term and long-term periods. Some expectations are easily identified, for example: that the service is of benefit to the student/client, that the programme operate at a reasonable cost, and that the programme improve. Other expectations are less obvious and may relate to methods of operation, image perception, location, and concerns that may remain unknown unless some effort is made to have the concerned groups clarify their expectations. The most important expectations should be reflected in the programme objectives and standards.

4. Agree on the purpose of the conjoint evaluation and what can be achieved. Is the evaluation being initiated to determine how closely the actual programme approximates the original model? Should the evaluation tell how the programme has improved or how various procedures have changed? Is the purpose of the conjoint evaluation to determine compliance with a specific mandate? Is the evaluation required to document whether additional funding should be authorized? There are many reasons why programmes are evaluated and the result usually involves making some kinds of judgement about the programme (Schalock, 1983). Whatever the reasons, they should be clearly stated and understood by the participants in the beginning, so that there is no doubt about the purpose.

A clearly articulated statement of purpose will provide direction for the evaluation and reports that are prepared. It would be unfortunate if some of the special interest groups expected the evaluation to provide information on some specific aspect of the programme or its service, but later found that this had not even been included in the evaluation purpose.

Of equal importance is how the conjoint evaluation will be used when the process is completed. The evaluators must know how the evaluation results will be used before they begin. This area is often poorly clarified and, therefore, can become the cause of fear and suspicion. Terms like evaluation, assessment, and examination tend to produce thoughts of danger and alarm in some people, but this uneasiness can be reduced and managed when there is agreement on the purpose and how the results will be used (Goldhammer, 1969). This should also include details on who will receive copies of the findings. In addition other individuals may be added to the list at a later stage, how will agreement be reached on their inclusion?

5. Determine the time and resources available. The evaluators must know what practical constraints exist on time and money before they can decide how extensive the evaluation should be. Knowing which resources they have at their disposal will affect the kind of data that can be collected, the methods used, the personnel involved, the frequency of meetings, etc. The evaluation design and schedule, in addition to projecting what can feasibly be accomplished when the evaluation goes according to plan, should also include contingency plans that can be implemented if something unforeseen occurs (Johnston et al., 1978).

6. Determine whose permission is required. This is an obvious point, but one that is easily overlooked. If permission is assumed to be available but is not when required, it can seriously damage the evaluation and be an embarrassment to the evaluators, and others involved (Fink & Kosecoff, 1980). Examples of the kinds of permission that may be required are:

- use of personal information that was given for another purpose. An example is the information provided in student/client application forms.
- use of resources and authorization to expend funds. Even though a programme may have a budget allocation for evaluation, authorization may still be required to initiate the process and to obtain the time and resources of other involved personnel. Although most

of the costs will likely be generated within the programme, there may also be resource implications for other programmes or agencies that will need approval.
- use of equipment and facilities. This may involve common meeting areas, recording equipment, and assessment instruments.

Whether permission to carry out various facets of a conjoint evaluation is a legal or ethical requirement, an obligation, or a common courtesy, it is seldom an area of difficulty if the process is well planned and the various special interest groups have been informed that their assistance and support may be needed.

7. Decide on the kind of data that can feasibly be collected. The evaluation questions will call for certain kinds of data, but can they be collected, and if so, what tools or approaches should be employed? Data can be collected by a number of common methods, for example, structured and unstructured interviews, surveys of participant and non-participant perceptions, student/client and programme records, behaviour observations, and personal assessments. The task of the evaluators is to adopt or design the instruments used to obtain the data required to answer the evaluation questions.
Because good quantifiable data about many aspects of human service programmes are difficult to obtain, personal assessments are often used as a source of information about programme quality and adequacy. Personal assessments are usually obtained from external evaluators, programme personnel, or other people with expertise. Subjective assessments despite their possible bias, can be a useful addition in supporting and enlarging upon quantifiable and other descriptive data.

8. Select the evaluation questions. People representing various programme interests whose views about the programme are considered important, should be involved in the process of selecting the evaluation questions. This is the time to involve the special interest groups who will not be involved in carrying out the evaluation. Some of these people may be unfamiliar with all aspects of the programme, and it will be necessary to take the time required to work through the process before reaching consensus on the most important questions. Remember, the final evaluation questions will determine the kind of data that will be collected.

Evaluation questions may be quite general or specific, for example:

- How have expenditures been translated into educational services?
- How responsible is the service to the individual needs of students?
- Which parts of the programme have shown the most improvement?

Before reaching agreement on the final set of evaluation questions, it is important to decide on the amount of effort that will be required to answer the questions and how the data will be collected. Some questions that initially sound very good may not be feasible if they are stated too generally, or if the time and resources available are inadequate to support using them. For example, an obvious question like: *What are the graduates doing now?* may be impossible to answer unless some mechanism exists to contact those who have moved or changed their addresses.

9. <u>Confirm the roles of the participants</u>. Once a decision is reached on what can feasibly be accomplished the participants can be assigned their tasks. Instructors, teachers and counsellors may already be collecting formative data as part of their regular work. Supervisors and others are often used to carry out time-samples and to initially collate data.

A major part of task assignment is to clarify who will be responsible for supervision of the process. It is very common for responsibility to be shared by the programme operator and the funding agency. Whatever the division of labour, it must be made clear to everyone involved to avoid possible confusion and to keep the evaluation on schedule (Fink & Kosecoff, 1984). The writer's experience is that it is most convenient for the programme operator to collect the evaluation data and for the funding agency to complete the data analysis and prepare the first draft of the final report. In order to ensure accountability, these tasks should be assigned to specifically designated people.

After taking care to address each of the foregoing points, and perhaps other issues of specific concern, the evaluation design should be complete. However, even with the best effort, it will not cover every possible eventuality. Even if this does happen, care should be taken to preserve the original purpose and general design, or a new evaluation approach will need to be developed with all of the associated time and resource costs.

IMPLEMENTATION PROCESS

The evaluation design stage addressed itself to *what* will be done. When it is completed, decisions about *how* the conjoint evaluation process will take place must be considered. There are a number of details to be monitored by the evaluators to ensure that the evaluation design is properly implemented. Some of the basic steps are:

1. Preparing the Evaluation Tools. Evaluation instruments and data collection forms can be adopted from commercial resources or developed by the programme. Some of the common kinds are:

   - surveys of perception and opinion that use a Likert-style format. (Van Dalen, 1979).
   - structured interview formats to give direction to the process.
   - formative data collection sheets which form part of the programme's regular feedback mechanism.
   - volume, behaviour, and opinion time-sampling.

2. Orienting the Participants and Assigning Responsibilities. Programme personnel and others assigned evaluation tasks should receive orientation and instruction. They should be familiar with: the reasons for using a conjoint evaluation approach, the project schedule, their responsibilities, task completion dates and the deadline for the final report.

3. Collecting the Data. The data collection stage may only take a week, or it may continue for several years, depending on the purpose and evaluation model used. During this stage, the project schedule should be closely monitored and feedback should be provided to keep participants informed on progress (Cook, 1971). If the evaluation has a large formative component, regular meetings with the participants should be held to review the evaluation process, condense the preliminary data, review interim reports and make programme modifications.

   Even when data collection forms are carefully prepared and personnel have been oriented to their tasks, the forms may still not be filled out properly. It is a good practice to regularly check data forms for completeness and accuracy as they are submitted. If checking is delayed until the data analysis stage, the missing data may no longer be retrievable. In addition, do not expect everyone to be as concerned as you are about the evaluation. This may seem obvious, but in practice, it is easy to overlook the fact that not everyone involved will necessarily agree that the programme should be evaluated. Occasionally it may be necessary to reassign individuals to other activities, if they do not fulfill their tasks adequately (Fink & Kosecoff, 1985).

DATA ANALYSIS AND REPORTING THE RESULTS

The primary task of evaluation is to determine changes which occurred in the students/clients, or in other specific goals as a result of the programme. The tasks of evaluators are much like those of detectives, collecting information from various sources to see if it supports possible explanations. Care must be exercised to ensure that all valid, supportive, or adverse information is used.

Some special steps should be taken in data analysis and preparation of the final report to reinforce the shared responsibilities that the evaluators have for the programme.

1. An outline of the proposed final report and any interim reports should be circulated to individuals that share responsibilities for the evaluation. This is a useful way to confirm the accuracy of the preliminary conclusions and to propose the content and structure of the final report. A large part of the conjoint evaluation process involves working together to learn as much as possible about the programme so that reasonable recommendations are made jointly. Information sharing strengthens the process and reduces the possibility that any of the participants will be surprised by the final results.

2. Since there are often several groups concerned about the programme, special consideration should be given to how the anticipated and unanticipated evaluation outcomes will affect the expectations held by the students/clients, the programme operator, the funding agency, and special interest groups. These expectations and the associated findings should be highlighted in the final report.

3. Even though a standard may exist, it is often very difficult to obtain good quantifiable data on some aspects of rehabilitation programmes. Personal perceptions and observations may be the only source of data available to explain what the programme did, but caution should be exercised since an over-reliance on qualitative data may seriously undermine the validity of the conclusions reached.

4. The various stages of programme maturation need to be carefully considered during data analysis. Since many

conjointly evaluated programmes are new, the formative and summative data will vary as the programme matures. This factor should be acknowledged and referred to in the findings.

5. It is often helpful to view a programme as a small system within a larger system. Any change, even in part of the programme, can potentially affect the overall programme and perhaps other programmes. The following is an example of some of the system questions that might be asked to focus the analysis:

   - Students/Clients. Has there been a change in the usual sources of applicants? Is the skill level of applications different than before?
   - Personnel. Has the availability of potential employees changed? Have the competencies required of personnel changed?
   - Employment market. Have there been any significant changes in the skill expectations of graduates?
   - Financial resources. Has the financial position of the programme changed? To what extent does the level of funding affect the soundness of programme development and management?

Normally the purpose of programme evaluation is to make some judgment about the merit, success, or worth of the programme. The findings usually flow from the initial evaluation questions and point to important outcomes in performance (quality and quantity), satisfaction (client and family), impact on others (services and people), personnel matters (turnover and skill level), improvement, and other issues. The conjoint evaluation process addresses these matters, but they are not the most important feature. The primary reason for using this approach is to bring the programme operator, the funding agency, and, to a degree, the interested parties, into a relationship that reinforces their mutual responsibilities and accountability for the programme and its services.

SOME RESULTS OF CONJOINT EVALUATION

There are a number of potential results from conjoint evaluation. Most of them are beneficial, but others have the potential of being problematic.

Benefits:

1. A major strength of the conjoint evaluation approach is that the process requires the evaluators to address

their mutual concerns about the programme and to take steps to ensure that the programme develops as completely as possible within existing constraints.

2. Since the conjoint evaluation process requires that the evaluation tasks be shared, there is a need for both the programme operator and the funding agency to understand the programme objectives, the expectations of the various concerned groups, and the evaluation process. This makes reaching conclusions about programme worth or future funding much less stressful, because the conclusions are jointly developed, based on information that is openly collected and analyzed. Both parties may initially start the evaluation process anticipating different outcomes, but at the conclusion they should not be surprised by the findings.

3. Since conjoint evaluation projects are normally carried out over a period of one to several years, there is usually ample opportunity to understand and to account for the effects that programme maturation can have on both formative and summative evaluation data.

4. Scheduling a conjoint evaluation over a significant period of time can encourage the development of a strong formative evaluation component. Regular individual and conjoint reviews of programme progress make it possible to adjust programme procedures based on ongoing experience. This can be a very helpful process in programme development.

5. Since information about the programme is conjointly gathered and analyzed by the evaluators, there is less reason for the programme operator or the funding agency to subjectively promote the programme. This high level of information sharing also appears to result in less suspicion by both parties about the motives of the other.

Potential Problems

1. The programme operator or the funding agency may lose sight of the fact that their primary responsibility is to the students/clients who need the service. Instead, their primary concern may focus on the future of the programme. The possibility of the results becoming biased can be minimized if the evaluation is well designed, the process is closely monitored, and interim reports are regularly circulated for review and comment.

2. The nature of human service programmes is such that value judgments about the adequacy of services often comprise a significant part of the evaluation.

Qualitative data should be analyzed as rigorously as possible to consider their quality based on the credibility, expertise, involvement, and self-interest of their source. Cross-checking data across several sources can reduce the effects of bias.

3. Although the programme operator and the funding agency will initially have agreed to work cooperatively, either party may attempt to disregard the agreement and attempt to achieve their separate and personal objectives. Examples of this are purposely providing inaccurate or incomplete data, selecting data that tends to support only a particular outcome, and preparing the final report without consultation or discussion. The possibility that these unacceptable actions could go unnoticed for long can be reduced by holding to the regularly scheduled progress reviews, circulating preliminary summaries and interim reports, and being willing to challenge information or procedures when in doubt.

4. If a conjoint evaluation agreement is discontinued or the cooperative approach becomes unworkable, then the additional costs of preparing another evaluation approach will be incurred. This can be minimized by careful preparation of the evaluation process, and by making the completion of a conjoint evaluation a condition of future funding or service availability.

This review of some of the potential benefits and problems of the conjoint evaluation model is not comprehensive, but it highlights a number of issues that programme operators or funding agencies should be aware of when considering programme evaluation. Most of the potential problems can be prevented or minimized by preplanning and a commitment by both parties to work together to provide the most effective and feasible service possible.

It would be an oversight to leave the reader with the impression that if programme operators and funding agencies would only carefully plan and share a commitment to provide the best possible service, then anticipated decisions about programme funding, or the value of their programme, would always be forthcoming and predictable. The conjoint evaluation process can be very helpful in refining programmes and preparing recommendations for individuals charged with responsibility for decision-making, but these are not the only ingredients that go into the approval process. Changes in service delivery, new priorities, potential choices, and available funding are variables outside the scope of conjoint evaluation, and they too are considered by decision-makers.

CONCLUSION

The evaluation process can be used for more than making judgments about the worth or effectiveness of programmes. It can also be used to improve and further develop programmes and services. In recent years the importance of accounting to a range of concerned groups for the effectiveness of social and educational programmes and the use of public and private funds has become widely expected. In some cases, it is required. This accountability is usually the responsibility of programme operators and funding agencies.

Programmes that provide services for persons with disabilities have expanded rapidly since the early 1970s. In most areas, recognized standards of performance have yet to be established. There is continuing pressure on funding agencies and programme operators from persons with disabilities and special interested groups for services to be extended and improved. There is good reason for programme operators and funding agencies to work together to define the kind and quality of services that should be provided. Conjoint evaluation can be a very effective evaluation approach in this environment because it reinforces a strong cooperative working relationship between the primary interest groups. It also focuses their attention on the service needs, the most effective kinds of programmes and those that are likely to work in the future. As we enter the next decade, it appears that there will be continuing pressure on programme operators and funding agencies to be more accountable for: a) provision of more effective programmes, b) greater integration between programmes within the service system, c) creation of recognized standards of practice, and d) the effective use of public and private resources.

Because rehabilitation is a developing service area, it is likely that there will also be an increasing and parallel demand for approaches that both judge programme effectiveness and provide a mechanism to assist responsible individuals and agencies further develop and refine the overall effectiveness of their services.

THE MAIN POINTS REVIEWED

1. A programme is traditionally evaluated to determine:
    a. If the service is required,
    b. Its effectiveness, and
    c. Its ability to meet individual and system needs.
2. Programme operators and funding agencies are primarily responsible for the provision of public services for persons with disabilities, and they both require

mechanisms that can provide accurate information about programme processes and outcomes.

3. Programmes for disabled persons are in a process of rapid evolution, and there are a number of special interest groups concerned about the effectiveness of the services provided.

4. Factors such as programme maturity and the expectations of special interest groups can strongly affect the kind of evaluation attempted and the results obtained.

5. The nine components of designing a conjoint evaluation are:
   a. Agreeing to evaluate conjointly.
   b. Agreeing on the purpose of the programme.
   c. Identifying the information needs of the interest groups.
   d. Agreeing on the purpose of the evaluation.
   e. Determining the resources available.
   f. Determining the permissions required.
   g. Deciding what data can be feasibly collected.
   h. Selecting the evaluation questions.
   i. Confirming the roles of the participants.

6. Implementing a conjoint evaluation process requires coordination. The various participants must be well informed, the schedule must be carefully monitored, and participants must fulfill their responsibilities if they are to benefit from the results and the information obtained.

7. The process of data analysis and preparation of a final report in conjoint program evaluation is similar to the same steps in other evaluation approaches. The major difference is the way that cooperative collection and analysis of the information reinforces the shared responsibilities that the programme operator and the funding agency have for the quality of services the programme provides.

REFERENCES

Accreditation Council for Services of Mentally Retarded and Other Developmental Disabled Persons (1980) 'Standards of Services for Developmentally Disabled Individuals,' *Accreditation Council, Washington, ix,* 59, 76.

Alberta Education (1985) *Report of the Minister's Advisory Committee: Foundation for the Future,* Alberta Education, Edmonton.

Beasley, D. M. G. (1984) 'Jack Tizard Memorial Lecture,' *Journal of Developmental Disabilities,* 10(3), 126-132.

Commission on Accreditation of Rehabilitation Facilities (1984) *Standards Manual,* Tucson, 10-20.

Cook, D. L. (1971) *Educational Project Management,* Charles
E. Merrill, Columbus.

DeJong, G. & Lifchez, R. (1983) 'Physical Disability and
Public Policy,' *Scientific American, 42.*

Elliot, R. (1980) 'Distributive Justice, Education and the
Handicapped,' in R. S. Laura (ed.), *Problems of
Handicap,* Macmillan Company of Australia PTY Ltd.,
South Melbourne.

Fink, A. & Kosecoff, J. (1980, 1984, 1985) *How to Evaluate
Educational Programs,* Capital Publications Inc.,
Arlington (April 1980 1-4 (2), September 1984, 1,
January 1985 2-4 (2).

Flynn, R. J. & Boschen, K. A. (1984) 'Program Evaluation in
Canadian Rehabilitation Services,' in N. J. Marlett, R.
Gall, and A. Wight-Felske (eds.), *Dialogue on
Disability: A Canadian Perspective,* The University of
Calgary Press, Calgary.

Frey, W. D. (1984) 'Functional Assessment in the '80's, in
A. S. Halpern & M. J. Fuhrer, (eds.), *Functional
Assessment in Rehabilitation,* Paul H. Brookes,
Baltimore.

Goldhammer, R. (1969) *Clinical Supervision,* Holt, Rinehart
and Winston, Inc., New York.

Johnston, C. P., Alexander, M. & Robin, J. (1978) *Quality
of Working Life: Evaluation and Measurement,* Labour
Canada, Ottawa, 1-6, 10-12 (2), 16, 21-30 (3).

Joint Committee on Standards for Education (1981) *Standards
for Evaluation of Educational Programs, Projects and
Materials,* McGraw-Hill, New York.

Kiernan, W. E. & Petzy, V. (1982) 'A Systems Approach to
Career and Vocational Educational Programs for Special
Needs Students,' in K. P. Lynch, W. E. Kiernan and J.
A. Stark (eds.), *Prevocational and Vocational Education
for Special Needs Youth,* Paul H. Brookes, Baltimore.

Schalock, R. L. (1983) *Services for Developmentally
Disabled Adults: Development, Implementation, and
Evaluation,* University Park Press, Baltimore.

Schmuck, R. A., Runkel, P. J., Arends, J. H. & Arends, R. I.
(1977) *The Second Handbook of Organizational
Development in Schools,* Mayfield Publishing Co., Palo
Alto.

Topliss, E. (1982) *Social Responses to Handicap,* Longman
Group Ltd., Essex.

Townsend, P. (1981) 'Employment and Disability,' in A.
Walker & P. Townsend (eds.), *Disability in Britain,*
Martin Robertson and Co. Ltd., Oxford.

Van Dalen, D. B. (1979) *Understanding Educational Research,*
McGraw-Hill, New York.

APPENDIX

Evaluation Design - 'Transitional/Vocational Programmes'

1.0 Overall Evaluation Design

    1.1 Definition of Purpose
    1.2 Definition of Terms

        1.2.1 Normalization
        1.2.2 Disabled/Handicapped

2.0 Overview of Programmes

    2.1 Objectives of the Programmes
    2.2 Description of the Programmes

3.0 Evaluation of the Programmes (by)

    3.1 Students in the Programmes
    3.2 Graduates of the Programmes
    3.3 Staff of the Programmes
    3.4 Drop-outs of the Programmes
    3.5 Employers of the Graduates
    3.6 Other Programme Personnel

4.0 Evaluation of Student Performance

    4.1 Course, Grades, etc.
    4.2 Employer ratings

5.0 Summary of Results by Group or Types of Programmes

6.0 Overall Findings of Programmes

7.0 Recommendations

Further details of the Evaluation Design and Procedure are available from the author.

Chapter Seven

A DEVELOPMENTAL SYSTEMS APPROACH TO PLANNING AND EVALUATING
SERVICES FOR PERSONS WITH HANDICAPS

David R. Mitchell

INTRODUCTION

From the moment when parents are first informed that their
child is handicapped, a life-long and life-wide process is
set in motion. The thesis of this chapter is that from the
point of initial diagnosis the planning, management and
evaluation of services for persons with handicaps should be
based on a developmental systems model (Mitchell, 1984,
1985). This model has two premises:

1)   that such services must take account of the
     ecology of the handicapped person's social
     environment,
2)   that they must be responsive to the changing
     developmental needs of the handicapped person and
     his or her family at various stages of the life
     cycle.

THE ECOLOGICAL PERSPECTIVE

Handicapped persons do not live in a social vacuum. All
have parents, most have siblings, and all exist in a society
with its particular mix of subcultures. From an ecological,
or systems, perspective, a family of a person with a handicap is seen as comprising an interpersonal system which, in
turn, is embedded in other systems of varying degrees of
remoteness from the family (Bristol & Gallagher, 1982;
Bronfenbrenner, 1979; Mitchell, 1984, 1985; Parke & Lewis,
1981; Pruchno, Blow & Smyer, 1984; Ramey, McPhee & Yates,
1982; Rubin & Quinn-Curran, 1983; Turnbull, Brotherson &
Summers, 1983). Specifically, as they affect a nuclear
family, these social systems comprise:

1) the <u>microsystem</u> of the family and its various subsystems;

2) the <u>mesosystem</u> with which the family members interact on a day-to-day basis (e.g. the extended family, specific health services, the school, the work setting);

3) the <u>exosystem</u> in which the mesosystem is embedded (e.g. the health system, the education system, voluntary agencies);

4) the <u>macrosystem</u>, made up of the broad values and beliefs that characterize the culture and subculture in which the family lives.

FIGURE 1   THE MAIN SYSTEMS OF RELEVANCE TO A FAMILY WITH A YOUNG HANDICAPPED CHILD

<u>Macrosystem</u>

1. Ethnic/Cultural
2. Socioeconomic
3. Religious
4. Economic
5. Political...

<u>Exosystem</u>

1. Mass media
2. Health
3. Voluntary Agencies
4. Social Welfare
5. Education...

<u>Mesosystem</u>

1. Medical and Health Workers
2. Extended Family
3. Friends/Neighbours
4. Work/Recreation Associates
5. Early Intervention Programmes
6. Other Parents
7. Parent Training Programmes
8. Local Community...

<u>Microsystem</u>

1. Mother-Father
2. Mother-Handicapped Child
3. Mother-Non-handicapped Child
4. Father-Handicapped Child
5. Father-Non-handicapped Child
6. Handicapped Child-Non-handicapped Child

Figure 1 presents a diagrammatic summary of the main components of a total system which are of relevance to a nuclear family made up of a mother and father, a handicapped child and his or her sibling.

The basic thesis of a systems approach as it applies to rehabilitation, then, is that the behaviour of a handicapped person cannot, and therefore must not, be considered in isolation from his or her social context. Or, as Bronfenbrenner (1979) has expressed it in relation to human development in general,

> '... the properties of the person and of the environment, the structures of the environmental settings, and the processes taking place within and between them must be viewed as interdependent and analyzed in systems terms.'

In meeting the needs of handicapped persons and their families consideration must be given to such factors as the transmission of information, the provision of support and the power relationships that exist in the interfaces between handicapped persons, their families, human service agencies and the broader society. For example, the welfare of a handicapped person is very dependent upon his or her parents accepting a prolonged period of dependence, a relationship that is dramatically different from that which usually pertains between parent and offspring, and one that is increasingly subject to scrutiny and challenge as handicapped persons' rights to self determination become accepted. A further example includes the continuous need of a family of a handicapped person for information on a range of topics, including their child's developmental potential, the services available in the community, and their legal entitlements. In turn, a family's capacity to cope with the problems presented by their handicapped child will be influenced by the attitudes and beliefs of the community in which they live and of the broader society.

The utility of this ecological approach to individuals and their families is not, of course, limited to persons with handicaps. Its principles have in part been derived from, and are certainly applicable to, all persons. There is a considerable and growing body of literature in which human development is construed as a bidirectional, reciprocal process which takes place in a family microsystem which, in turn, has reciprocal relationships with its sociocultural milieu (Bell & Harper, 1977; Brazelton, Koslowski & Main, 1974; Bronfenbrenner, 1979; Clarke-Stewart, 1978; Feiring & Lewis, 1978; Lewis and Feiring, 1980; Lytton, 1980; Parke, 1978; Parke & Lewis, 1981).

The Nature of Systems

Since one of the principal assumptions of this chapter is that a systems approach to planning and evaluating services for handicapped persons has high utility, the following discussion presents a brief outline of the main character-istics of systems.

Wholeness: Although structurally a system is made up of a set of subsystems (as noted earlier), these elements must comprise a whole for the term system to apply. Thus Ackoff and Emery (1972) used the phrase *set of interrelated elements*, while Hare, (1967) wrote of an *holistic orientation*. In the field of services for handicapped persons, for example, one might ask if the health education, and welfare services form part of a whole human services system, along with the families of handicapped persons, or are they a series of separate, and even competing systems (Mitchell, 1978)?

Connectedness. If a set of elements comprise a whole, they must, of course, be connected in some significant way. While in a sense everything is connected to everything, elements make up a system only when certain criteria are met. Chief among these is the notion of connectedness or interrelatedness (Ackoff & Emery, 1972; Broderick & Smith, 1979; Feiring & Lewis, 1978; Miller, 1978; Mitchell, 1978; Stewart et al., 1978; von Bertalanffy, 1968). The fact that a system comprises a set of interrelated elements leads us to the important point that a system is characterized not only by the nature of its elements, but also by the multiple interactions that occur between and among those elements. This latter feature, known as the principle of non-summativity, is what is meant when it is claimed that the whole is more than the sum of its parts. Thus the behaviour of a family system is not limited to the actions of its members, but must encompass the interactions between and among them.

Range of stability. According to Miller (1978) and Ramey, McPhee and Yates (1982), each variable within a system has a range of stability that is maintained in equilibrium (albeit constantly changing) by transactions within the system and between the system and its environ-ment. This notion of equilibrium, or more accurately *steady state* (Feiring & Lewis, 1978) in turn leads to the cybernetic principle that a successful system must have a mechanism for sensing perturbations and for regulating its behaviour to maintain a desired relationship between input and output (Griffiths, 1964; Pratt, 1982). In cybernetic terms, this requires that a feedback loop of some kind operates to maintain the system within its desired range of stability. Any variable that forces the system beyond this range constitutes a stressor which has to be dealt with, otherwise the system disintegrates. The extent to which a family system is able successfully to deal with the potential stressor of a handicapped person depends on a variety of factors which will be dealt with later in this chapter.

The Family Microsystem

When viewed from a systems perspective which embraces the whole of human society, the family of a handicapped person is seen as comprising a microsystem in which various activities, roles, and reciprocal interpersonal relationships are experienced between the handicapped person and his or her parents and siblings. In western cultures, the family microsystem typically comprises three major subsystems (Minuchin, 1974):

> The spouse subsystem (i.e., husband-wife interactions),
> The parental subsystem (i.e., parent-child interactions), and
> The sibling subsystem (i.e., child-child interactions).

The number of reciprocal relationships (R) subsumed under these three subsystems depends, of course, on the number of members in a family (M), according to the following formula:

$$R = \frac{M(M-1)}{2}$$ (Broderick and Smith, 1979).

Thus, in a family comprising a mother, a father, and two children, there are six possible reciprocal relationships. Not only does the number of relationships increase as family size increases, but also, as Feiring and Lewis (1978) have pointed out, indirect or *second-order*, influences become possible. This point was taken up by Turnbull, Brotherson and Summers (1983) when they argued that healthy family life involves a complex balancing of individual and group interests in which equal importance should be accorded to the well-being of every family member. They illustrate how this balance can be disrupted when a mother works with a handicapped child on a feeding programme during the family mealtime. While she is doing so, her availability for interactions with other members of the family are correspondingly reduced. As well, there may be consequential negative effects on future interactions involving the handicapped child and others in the family because of resentment generated by the handicapped child's taking so much of the mother's attention. To reiterate an earlier point: at the core of the systems approach is the notion of multiple interactions among elements, with the behaviour of any one element being influenced by the behaviours of other elements in the system.

The implication of this perspective for the planning and evaluation of services for handicapped persons is quite simply that intervention must at least take the dynamics of the family microsystem into account; better still, it should be directed at the total microsystem. Research and services have recently shown an increased appreciation of the family ecology of handicap, with an encouraging awareness of interactions between handicapped persons, their parents (including fathers), and their siblings. Representative of intervention aimed at helping parent-child interactions to become more reciprocal and more mutually pleasurable is the work of Bromwich (1981), Field (1979), and Field et al. (1980), all of whom have worked with pre-term babies and their parents, mainly mothers. The notion of dyad-focused programmes, however, is equally applicable to handicapped persons. Although, as McConachie (1982) and Lamb (1983) have pointed out, research into the involvement of fathers with handicapped children is quite sparse - and is almost exclusively focused on the fathers of mentally handicapped children - this is slowly changing and the next few years will probably see an increasing responsiveness to the needs of fathers of handicapped persons. Research into the relationship between handicapped persons and their siblings has similarly been neglected, but here, too, there are the beginnings of a foundation on which intervention programmes could be based (Grossman, 1972; Kew, 1975; Parfit, 1975; Seligman, 1983; Simeonsson & McHale, 1981; Skrtic et al., 1983).

The Mesosystem

Just as a handicapped person interacts with other members of his or her family microsystem, so, too, does the family interact with its wider social context, or its mesosystem. This is made up of the *extra-familial* (Minuchin, 1974) systems in which the family members, either collectively or individually, actively participate as they go about their daily lives. For a family with a handicapped member, the mesosystem typically includes the extended kinship groups, friends and neighbours, work and recreation associates, other families with a handicapped member, the local community, and the host of statutory and voluntary agencies involved in delivering services to handicapped persons. As noted by Parke and Lewis (1981), these influences are bidirectional and can be either positive or negative.

Services for handicapped persons and their families must help them deal with these mesosystem elements. This process of negotiating what Rubin and Quinn-Curran (1983) refer to as a *massive maze* is by no means easy, particularly when the maze may lack the attributes of wholeness and connectedness. Helping parents to obtain information and support from the various mesosystem elements and to be able to make significant inputs into the mesosystem comprises a very legitimate goal for professionals working with handicapped persons. Similarly, the task of acquainting the extended family and friends and associates of the family with the needs of handicapped persons is one that should not be overlooked.

The Exosystem

The mesosystem is, in turn, embedded in an exosystem. At this level, consideration is given to the various formal and informal organizations present in society which, through their procedures, regulations and value systems, have a bearing on a family with a handicapped member. This impact is generally indirect and mediated by individuals or organizations at the mesosystem level. Included in the exosystem, then, are the health, employment, education, social welfare, recreation, voluntary societies, and mass media systems.

The elements of the exosystem have a significant, albeit indirect, bearing upon the way a family perceives and interacts with its handicapped member and on the ways in which systems at the mesosystem level interact with the family. The mass media, for example, can be quite powerful in creating or transmitting attitudes towards handicapped persons, as two recent examples in New Zealand testify. Firstly, there is the image of handicap as reflected in a series of telethon appeals - an image of disability rather than of ability, of grace-and-favour charity rather than of rights, and of *cuteness* rather than of reality. And, secondly, although there have been considerable improvements in recent years, the media seem to have a penchant for publicizing the *magic* of esoteric cures as, for example, in the recent attention given to a mother's unverified claims of her 3½ year-old Down's Syndrome daughter *reading from books for primary school children that had been translated into five languages* and *delving into the mysteries of square roots and fractions* (N.Z. Herald, July 29, 1983).

Since the health system is one of the early elements of the exosystem to impinge on a family, it is important that attention be given to its collective ethos. The medical model, with its focus on disabilities and causation and on

the physical care of handicapped persons - often in institutional settings - has been antithetical to a developmental
model in which the emphasis is on building on strengths
through community care, socialization and education, and on
community care.

The education system is another exosystem element which
has a major impact on the way in which a family perceives
its handicapped member. Like the health system, it is
undergoing a rapid series of changes, with the emphasis
shifting from a *separate but equal* model of services for
handicapped children to an integrationist model based on
such principles as zero reject, least restrictive environments, and preparation for living in the community.
Clearly, these philosophies, as manifested in the special
education provisions, will affect a family's expectations
for, and interactions with, its handicapped member.

On the basis of the systems approach presented in this
chapter, it is suggested that it may be just as appropriate
for professionals to bring about changes in the exosystem as
it is to work with individual families. This may mean, for
example, making conscious attempts to educate media representatives and to influence the various statutory and
voluntary agencies into adopting more enlightened approaches
towards handicapped persons and their families. In short,
the best service may sometimes take the form of advocacy on
behalf of those with handicaps. At the very least, it
should take account of the impact of the exosystem on the
families of handicapped persons.

The Macrosystem

And, finally, there is the macrosystem, made up of the broad
values, beliefs and ideologies that characterize a society.
These influences may be broadly grouped under such headings
as ethnic/cultural, socioeconomic, religious, economic, and
political - all of which have an indirect but significant
impact on a family with a handicapped person. The ideologies of the systems at this level are frequently unexam-
ined, mainly because they are taken for granted or are below
the consciousness of the people. Also, because the
prevailing ideologies underpin the power-base of those
exercising control over society, attempts to challenge them
are frequently suppressed.

How then does the macrosystem impact the family of a
handicapped person? Factors such as ethnicity, religion and
socioeconomic status - all of which spring from the macro-
system - seem to act as broad predictors of a family's
reactions to a handicapped member. A society's prevailing
political and economic ideologies are other macrosystem
variables which have a major impact on persons with

handicaps in such areas as the levels of financial assistance available for benefits, the recognition of human rights and employment opportunities. Here again, professionals must not only take prevailing ideologies into account in their work, but they must also accept some responsibility for bringing about changes where such ideologies are antithetical to the welfare of handicapped persons and their families. The fact that these ideologies are deeply embedded in society and are the source of great sensitivity when they are raised, should not be a deterrent. In the last analysis, a political stand is taken whether one seeks to bring about structural change in society or goes along with the prevailing ideology. There is no middle ground.

Adapting to Persons with Handicaps

Earlier in this chapter, reference was made to the range of stability possessed by a system and how the family microsystem must evolve coping strategies or face the threat of disintegration. While it is possible to detect broad trends from the literature on families of handicapped persons, it is abundantly clear that particular individuals and particular families have unique reactions to handicap (Challela, 1981). Just as some seem to benefit from their association with a handicapped person in the family, some seem to have their development put at risk. Thus, some marriages seem to be strengthened, while others are placed in jeopardy (Howard, 1978; Lamb, 1983; McConachie, 1982; Price-Bonham & Addison, 1978; Wikler, 1981). Similarly, while some siblings appear to derive benefits from having a handicapped brother or sister, others do not and may even be psychologically harmed by the experience (Parfit, 1975; Seligman, 1983; Simeonsson & McHale, 1981; Skrtic et al., 1983). Further, as Hewett (1970) and Mittler and Mittler (1982) caution, we should beware of drawing too sharp a distinction between families of handicapped and non-handicapped persons; they have more in common with each other than is often recognized.

A useful framework for conceptualizing the factors that influence a family's response to handicap, based on the writings of Hill (1949), Burr (1973), McCubbin et al. (1980), and Turnbull, Brotherson and Summers (1983), is presented in Figure 2.

From this model, it can be seen that the extent to which the presence of a handicapped person in a family creates stresses is dependent upon many interacting conditions. At the broadest level, three factors determine a family's vulnerability to stress.

FIGURE 2 FACTORS THAT INFLUENCE A FAMILY'S RESPONSE TO HANDICAP

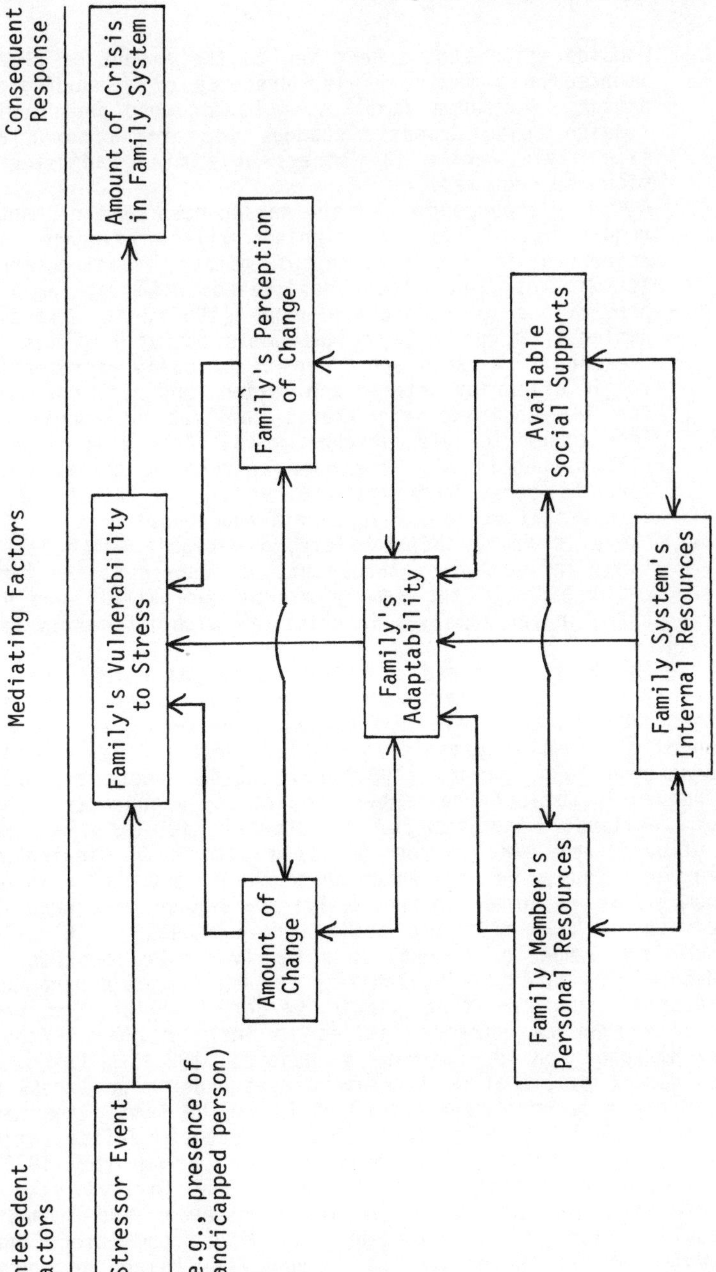

Antecedent Factors

Mediating Factors

Consequent Response

Stressor Event

(e.g., presence of handicapped person)

Family's Vulnerability to Stress

Family's Perception of Change

Amount of Change

Family's Adaptability

Available Social Supports

Family Member's Personal Resources

Family System's Internal Resources

Amount of Crisis in Family System

1. Consideration should be given to the amount of change imposed on a family by the presence of a handicapped person. For some families, a handicapped person will require quite dramatic changes in earning power and life style, while for others only minor adjustments might be required.

2. A family's perception of the seriousness of the changes required in its functioning will influence its responses to its handicapped member. Socioeconomic status has long been associated with a family's perceptions of handicap, Farber (1962), for example, noting that for high socioeconomic status families the presence of a handicapped person typically represents a tragic disparity between aspirations and reality, while for low socioeconomic status families it requires a less traumatic role reorganization. According to Reiss (1981), people with the same culture or social class tend to agree with one another on the magnitude of stress that various life events engender.

3. There is family adaptability, a variable which is, in turn, influenced by three sets of resources, the first two reside in the family microsystem itself and the third in the family's interactions with its mesosystem.

The first of these comprise the personal resources of each family, particularly their educational accomplishments, their health, and their self esteem. The second set is made up of the family system's internal resources. As Turnbull, Brotherson and Summers (1983) have noted, these resources frequently reflect the membership and style characteristics of families. The size of the family, for example, can influence the way in which it adapts to a handicapped member. Thus, there is evidence to the effect that a larger number of children in a family can reduce the negative effects of a handicapped child (Trevino, 1979). Clearly, too, the number of parents in a family can be important in determining parental availability for working on programmes. Research suggests that single parent families are more likely than two-parent families to institutionalize their handicapped child (German & Maisto, 1982). There is evidence, too, that mothers are placed under more stress by the presence of a handicapped child in the family than are fathers (Wilkin, 1979; Wing, 1975), but that marital satisfaction helps alleviate this stress (Friedrich, 1979). Religious commitment also influences the family system's internal resources. In Turnbull, Brotherson and Summers' (1983) study, for example, religious commitment was mentioned with unanticipated frequency as being the source of important coping strategies for parents. Family adaptability is also conditioned by a third set of resources available to it, namely the amount and quality of the informal and formal social supports available to it from the mesosystem level of the community (Friedrich & Friedrich, 1981; Howard, 1978; Parke & Lewis, 1981; Suelzle & Keenan, 1981).

THE LIFE-CYCLE PERSPECTIVE

Just as human service professionals should think of handicapped persons as living in social contexts, so too should they think of these contexts as changing over time. The second assumption of the developmental systems approach, then, is that families typically develop through a life-cycle. Although this life-cycle approach to family analysis has a long history in family sociology (Alpert, 1981; Nock, 1982), it has only recently been applied systematically to families of handicapped persons (Mitchell, 1985; Rubin & Quinn-Curran, 1983; Skrtic et al., 1983; Suelzle & Keenan, 1981; Turnbull, Brotherson & Summers, 1983; Wikler, Wasow & Hatfield, 1981).

From the life-cycle perspective, families are considered to pass through a series of stages related to the development of the handicapped person, each of which is characterized by a set of *developmental tasks* (Havighurst, 1972). These tasks result from interactions within the microsystem of the family, as well as from interactions between the family and the social systems in which it is embedded. While many of these tasks are common to all families as they assist in the development of their members, others are quite specific to the families of a handicapped person. It is argued that these tasks have to be at least partially mastered if families are to reach a satisfactory equilibrium in adapting to the stresses associated with the presence of a handicapped person (O'Hara, Chaiklin & Mosher, 1980; Seligman, 1979; Simeonsson & Simeonsson, 1981; Suelzle & Keenan, 1981). As a corollary, human service agencies should offer assistance that is appropriate not only to the changing developmental needs of handicapped persons as they grow older, but also to the changing needs of the family over its life cycle.

Changes in the life cycle are bounded by what Wikler (1981) terms *transition points*. These occur when there is a major discrepancy between expected (or idealized) achievement and actual performance and/or when there are major changes in service delivery systems. An example of the former is when parents are first informed that their child is handicapped or at risk - a point at which many parents feel a sense of grief for the death of their hoped-for child. The latter type of transition occurs, for example, when a child commences school or when he or she finishes school and enters into an occupation or some form of

137

sheltered employment. Using these criteria, it is possible to identify four broad stages in the life cycle of a family with a handicapped member when the initial diagnosis is made at or near birth (see also Brown & Hughson, 1980):

1.   Initial diagnosis,
2.   Infancy and toddlerhood,
3.   Childhood and early adolescence,
4.   Late adolescence and adulthood.

THE DEVELOPMENTAL SYSTEMS PERSPECTIVE

The ecological and life-cycle perspectives described above come together to make up the developmental systems approach. In planning and evaluating services for persons with handicap, each perspective is necessary; one without the other is insufficient for it will lead to inappropriately narrow programmes.

This section will examine the range of developmental tasks that confront the family microsystem as it interacts with its surrounding mesosystem, exosystem and macrosystem during the four stages outlined above. In considering these developmental tasks, certain assumptions will be made: that the reference point is an intact nuclear family, that the handicapped person has a non-handicapped sibling of a similar age, that the presence of a handicapping condition was detected at or near birth, and that the family sub-scribes to a broad western value system. In practice, of course, only some or even none of these assumptions might be appropriate, an eventuality that administrators and professionals who work with families must take into account.

Developmental Tasks at the Time of Initial Diagnosis

In this early phase, when the parents are first informed that their child is handicapped or at risk for handicap, a series of tasks begins to unfold. Some of these tasks are unique to this stage; others remain as a constant backdrop to living with a handicapped family member. Some are confronted in the hospital or perhaps in the doctor's surgery almost within minutes of the diagnosis; others only become apparent when the family as a whole in its home and community begins to come to terms with the reality of handicap. Some involve the spouse subsystem; some involve the parental subsystem; some impinge on the sibling sub-system; still others are deeply personal and private, touching the inner subjective world of the mother or the father.

The following represent some of the most important tasks confronting families of handicapped children during this stage, together with the implications for service planning:

a) <u>Deciding whether to pursue aggressive medical care when the infant's life is at risk.</u> It is unfortunate, but true, that one of the first tasks some parents have to face in their interactions with the mesosystem is such a complex ethical, legal and medical issue. This task confronts many parents of infants with severe congenital anomalies such as spina bifida, cardiac defects, hydrocephalus and duodenal atresia. In the recent past, there was a willingness on the part of medical personnel to permit parents not to elect surgery in such cases, or even to take unilateral decisions to withhold life-saving treatment (Duff & Campbell, 1973; Todres, et al., 1977). The current trend, however, is to support the 1971 United Nations Declaration on the Rights of Mentally Handicapped Persons which stated, *inter alia*, that mentally handicapped persons have a right to proper medical care (see, for example, Guess et al., 1984; Hardman, 1984; Mittler, 1984; President's Commission for the Study of Ethical Problems in Medicine and Biomedical and Behavioural Research, 1983; Raye & Healey, 1984, Shearer, 1985). Thus, several of the main US and Canadian organizations concerned with handicap have recently (1983-84) endorsed a comprehensive set of principles for the treatment of disabled infants. Their statement included the following: *Discrimination of any type against any individual with a disability/disabilities, regardless of the nature or severity of the disability, is morally and legally indefensible.* Parents should therefore be acquainted with the legal and ethical ramifications of their decisions to give or withhold consent for treatment.

b) <u>Deciding whether to keep the child in the family or to seek institutionalization or adoption.</u> In recent years, there has been a distinct trend in western societies for handicapped persons to be maintained in their families and in the community, rather than being institutionalized (Annison & Young, 1980; Bayley, 1973; Bruininks et al., 1980; Wilkin, 1979). This is not to say, however, that individual parents of handicapped or at-risk infants have sufficient contact with the field of disability to be aware of current practices. As with the previous task, human service agencies must take account of parents' needs for information and expert counselling relating to this task, not only from medical personnel, but also from social workers and psychologists who are in a position to talk about future prospects for them and their child and are recognized as expert witnesses in a wide range of legal systems. Both this and the previous task also involve helping parents to develop personal ideologies to guide their decision-making (Turnbull, Brotherson & Summers, 1983).

c) Accepting the reality of the handicapping condition. While this task is one that never ends, important steps along this path are made by many parents during these early days. Featherstone (1981), in her sensitive and intelligent account of family life, sees acceptance as comprising four processes:

1) acknowledging the existence of the handicap and its long-term significance,
2) integrating the child and the disability into the family,
3) learning to forgive their own errors and shortcomings, and
4) searching for meaning in their loss.

During this initial stage, the first of these processes is the pre-eminent task. Another factor that should be taken into account is that fathers and mothers appear to have different approaches to the reality of a handicap, fathers responding less emotionally and focusing on possible long-term problems and mothers responding more emotionally and expressing concerns about their ability to cope with the burdens of child care (Lamb, 1983). Counselling therefore needs to involve both parents.

d) Comprehending the nature of the handicap, its causation and its developmental possibilities. This developmental task translates into an obligation on the part of service agencies to provide families with accurate information on the nature of handicapping conditions and on available support services. Such information should be sensitively conveyed, preferably to both parents together with written supplementation and ample opportunities for follow-up interviews (Cunningham & Sloper, 1977; Gayton & Walker, 1974; Hornby, in press; Lonsdale, 1978; Mitchell, 1981a; Mittler & Mittler, 1982; Spain & Wigley, 1975). Since the medical profession bears the main responsibility for informing parents of their child's handicap (Mitchell, 1981a) it is important that its members accept responsibility for becoming well informed and skilled in helping parents cope with this task (Gayton, 1975; Lipton & Svarstad, 1977; Sanson-Fisher & Maguire, 1980; Wolraich & Reiter, 1979).

e) Maintaining or enhancing one's usual self concept. According to Featherstone (1981), this task is especially

applicable to mothers. She argues that since the whole
culture supports a mother in the opinion that her children
are what she has made them, she is particularly vulnerable
to a diminished sense of achievement and self-esteem and a
heightened sense of guilt when a child is handicapped.
While there is evidence that by no means all parents suffer
a diminution of self concept (Dunlap & Hollingsworth, 1977;
Gallagher, Cross & Scharfman, 1981; Guess et al., 1984), it
is clear that professionals who work with families at this
stage should be competent in helping parents reconstruct
their sense of identity where necessary (Hornby, in press;
Seligman, 1979).

f) Maintaining or enhancing one's relationships with
one's spouse. As noted earlier in this chapter, the
presence of a handicapped person in the family seems to
strengthen some marriages and jeopardize others. The
precise impact of handicap on the spouse subsystem is
determined by a complex amalgam of mediating factors, as
outlined in Figure 2, and requires sensitive analysis by
family workers if the appropriate kind of support is to be
given. Nevertheless, it is generally true that at this
stage of initial diagnosis parents must *receive* support from
parents, friends, siblings and professionals from the
mesosystem if they are to develop the resources to *give*
support to each other (Featherstone, 1981).

g) Understanding and coming to terms with the
reactions of the extended family, friends and associates.
On some occasions, professionals might quite deliberately
have to assist families to reestablish links with their
natural networks in the face of what appears to be abandon-
ment, but is often no more than bewilderment (Challela,
1981; Rubin & Quinn-Curran, 1983). Helping the important
people in this natural network to come to terms with their
reactions to handicap and to the family subsystem may well
be an important part of this process.

h) Establishing a positive parenting relationship with
the handicapped infant. While this task makes heavy demands
on both parents, it is one that fathers can find particularly difficult, mainly because they have fewer opportunities for physical and psychological contact (Featherstone,
1981; McConachie, 1982).

i) Maintaining or enhancing relationships between
parents and their non-handicapped children. With the
turmoil of adjusting to a handicapped child, parents often
find themselves lacking in emotional energy or time to
attend to the needs of their non-handicapped children, or
they may over-compensate and become too deeply dependent on

141

them, seeking emotional satisfactions they feel their handicapped child will deny them (Skrtic, et al., 1983).

Developmental Tasks During Infancy and Toddlerhood

Merging into the previous stage is the stage of infancy and toddlerhood, characterized by a broadening of the contacts with various mesosystem groups or agencies. During this period, the parents become more directly involved in the practical and developmental aspects of coping with a handi-capped child. The emotional issues that were dominant in the earlier stage are still present in many families and may reappear, but typically the parents now begin to look beyond the family and ask of themselves and of others in the mesosystem: *How can we best help our child and our family?* During this stage, then, tasks such as the following emerge:

a) Becoming familiar with and accessing appropriate support services provided by the various statutory and voluntary agencies. In most western societies, this means dealing with a wide range of services, including early intervention programmes, social work agencies, health services and welfare agencies. Because these agencies are frequently uncoordinated and are sometimes even in competi-tion with each other, parents can find the task of obtaining access to the appropriate services a difficult one. An important goal of professionals who work with families at this stage, then, is to help parents obtain adequate information on what is available and to acquire the basic communication and organizational skills that are necessary if they are to avail themselves of the services they need and to which they are entitled (Rubin & Quinn-Curran, 1983). Professionals must therefore have a thorough knowledge of agencies and services that are available in their communities.

b) Establishing a profitable working relationship with particular professionals. The parent-professional relationship varies from one where the parent has minimal communication with the professional, with both carrying out their functions in isolation from each other, through one where the parent acts as an aide or agent of the profes-sional, carrying out the latter's instructions, to one where there is a true, two-way partnership based on mutual respect. The third of these relationships seems to offer the most fruitful utilization of the unique skills, perceptions and experiences of parents and professionals (Mitchell, 1982; Mittler & Mittler, 1982).

142

c) <u>Making contact with other families</u>. Research suggests that the overwhelming majority of parents of handicapped children place a high value on meeting parents of children with similar handicaps (Carr, 1975; Mitchell, 1981b). Professionals should facilitate such contacts, but in doing so should recognize that a significant minority (15 per cent in Mitchell's 1981b study) want nothing to do with other parents or would prefer to take their time in making contacts, particularly in the early stages of working through their feelings. The recent growth of group counseling (Hornby, in press; Meyerson, 1983) and of parent-to-parent support networks (Mitchell, 1983(a)) testifies to the benefits many parents feel they derive from meeting with others with similar problems and experiences.

d) <u>Coping with the reactions of the broader community</u>. In the earlier stage, the families of a handicapped person had to adjust to their extended family, friends and associates. In this stage, the process of *coming out* is extended into the broader mesosystem settings as the family interacts with shopkeepers, people on buses, strangers at a sports event, and a host of others. These interactions frequently call upon competence in dealing with the uncomfortable social transactions that result from people's inexperience in dealing with handicaps. Families may need professional help in developing effective strategies and counselling in dealing with the anger and confusion that will result from unsuccessful transactions.

e) <u>Establishing a *balanced* family and personal life</u>. While the notion of balance is personal and unique to each family microsystem, most would agree that families should avoid the extreme positions of enmeshment or disengagement with the handicapped child (Skrtic, et al., 1983). Professionals can best help families in this regard by focusing on goal clarification rather than seeking to prescribe values.

f) <u>Developing competence in facilitating the handicapped child's development and in coping with the practical, day-to-day tasks of caring for him or her</u>. As McConachie 1982) has pointed out, this task may pose particular problems to fathers who may have little experience in playing with children during this period. This task also raises the question of how far parents can be expected to take on the roles of being their child's teacher, without jeopardizing the essential elements of being a parent (Katz, 1980).

g) <u>Coping with the developmental needs of the non-handicapped children in the family</u>. As Parfit (1975) has noted, resentment of parental attention to the handicapped child is a common phenomenon among non-handicapped siblings and this can become a problem during this stage, as can parental over-reliance on the non-handicapped siblings to act as the handicapped child's playmate (Skrtic et al., 1983).

Developmental Tasks During Childhood and Early Adolescence

During this stage, in addition to the various agencies from the previous stage that continue to be of relevance, the handicapped child and his or her family come in contact with an increasing range of settings at the mesosystem level. Chief among the new settings is the special education system, but also of importance are the various recreational and work experience settings, particularly as the child grows older. Respite services provided in some countries also play a prominent role for some families. This stage is usually finished when the handicapped person moves from a special educational to a vocational setting and, in some cases, from living at home to a residential facility of some kind.

The main developmental tasks facing families during this stage, and their implications for service delivery, are as follows:

a) _Participating in decisions relating to special education._ Recent trends in special education suggest that as a minimum this participation should include consultation with parents (Strickland, 1983), but should also embrace the notion of the parent-professional partnership (Mittler & McConachie, 1983; Mittler & Mittler, 1982) developed in the previous stage. The importance of parent participation in special education is clearly recognized, for example, in the United States' Education of All Handicapped Children Act of 1975 (PL94-142) and in the United Kingdom's 1981 Education Act (Mitchell, 1983b).

If parents are to avail themselves of these rights to participate in decisions involving their child's special education, or to obtain them when they are not present, they may well require assistance in developing appropriate communication and advocacy skills to deal with professional educators. If for no other reason than to make the special education system comprehensible to parents, efforts should be made, too, to coordinate its various subsystems (Mitchell, 1978).

b) _Accepting the prolonged dependence of the handicapped child._ While most children are rapidly acquiring social, physical and intellectual skills during this stage, the parents of a child with a handicap become increasingly aware of the child's limitations as more and more of society's hurdles seem impossible or, at best, difficult to accomplish. As these discrepancies with average rates of development become increasingly apparent during this stage, there may well be tendency for parents to become resistant towards the normalization concept (Suelzle & Keenan, 1981).

c) Helping the handicapped child and the community to adapt to each other. At one level, this task involves conscious efforts to educate the public as to the nature of handicapping conditions and the rights of persons with handicaps, while at another level it involves helping the handicapped child to understand his or her handicap and to develop social skills in dealing with other people's reactions.

d) Placing reasonable responsibilities on non-handicapped children for the care of their handicapped sibling. During this stage, the non-handicapped brother and sister (particularly the latter) are increasingly likely to be recruited as participants in the task of caring for their handicapped sibling (Seligman, 1983; Skrtic et al., 1983). Unless handled very carefully, this can be the source of resentment. On the other hand, it can be an enriching experience for, as Simeonsson and McHale (1981) have pointed out, siblings of handicapped children are often character-ized by a maturity and a responsible attitude that goes beyond their age.

e) Helping the non-handicapped sibling to develop strategies for explaining handicap to their peers. In view of the trend towards integrating handicapped children into regular school environments, it is increasingly likely that they will attend the neighbourhood school along with their non-handicapped siblings. Helping the latter to explain handicap and to understand the reactions of other children and teachers, both to themselves and their handicapped sibling, therefore becomes an important counselling goal.

Developmental Tasks During Late Adolescence and Adulthood

Just as attitudes towards and provisions for handicapped children have undergone profound changes in recent years, so too have changes impinged upon handicapped adolescents and adults and their families. In view of the fact that many of these changes have taken place during the life cycle of contemporary parents of handicapped adults, it is a pity that there is very little research available on this group (Mittler & Mittler, 1982). One might speculate, however, that during this stage many parents experience difficulty in adjusting their old ways of thinking about their handicapped children to modern ideas on the rights of handicapped persons. As noted by Mittler and Mittler (1982) *parents of adolescents and young adults have often reached a modus vivendi and a quality of adjustment to their situation which needs to be respected and which is in any case not easily changed.*

During this stage, the family microsystem typically undergoes major structural changes as the non-handicapped siblings leave home and as the handicapped person takes on increasing independence, even to the extent of pursuing a life outside of his or her family origin. And, of course, the parents eventually die. Major changes take place, too, in the type of agencies at the mesosystem level with which the handicapped person and his or her family interact. The school system no longer plays a dominant role and is replaced with work and/or long-term residential settings, typically operated in western societies by non-government voluntary agencies. Rubin and Quinn-Curran (1983) liken the school to a gatekeeper and monitor of their child's services. For many families school learning is regarded as being *tantamount to falling into an abyss.* Services for young adults, they claim, suffer from a greater degree of fragmentation than those for school-aged children.

Several developmental tasks confront the families of handicapped persons during their late adolescence and adulthood; these must be taken into account in the planning and administration of services.

a) <u>Adapting to the handicapped person's needs for dependence/independence.</u> This task involved accepting that while the handicapped person has a right to enjoy maximum independence, they will continue to have dependency needs which might have to be met by the family. The latter needs require an emotional adjustment to the chronicity of the handicapping condition (Turnbull, Brotherson & Summers, 1983) and may sometimes involve assuming a full-time care role (Mittler & Mittler, 1982), a role that greatly inhibits parents from moving on to the next stage of personal development that parents of non-handicapped children can normally aspire to (Rubin & Quinn-Curran, 1983). The other end of the continuum, accepting that the handicapped person may wish to live outside the family home, can be equally demanding for parents to adjust to. Whatever the balance of dependence or independence that is appropriate to the particular family, Mittler and Mittler (1982) feel that teaching social independence and community living skills constitutes one of the most important and distinctive roles of parents and families during this stage.

b) <u>Understanding and accepting the handicapped person's sexuality and possible wish for close and enduring relationships outside the family.</u> This task may even include families coming to accept the notion that the handicapped person may wish to marry and have children. A good deal of work has been done in recent years to help handicapped persons understand their rights and options in the field of human relationships (Johnson, 1984), but rather less has been done to help parents and non-handicapped siblings to develop philosophies and strategies to assist the handicapped person to obtain fulfillment in this area.

c) <u>Becoming familiar with and helping the handicapped person to pursue his or her legal rights.</u> As a result of the very recent emergence of concern among human service professionals and legal experts for the rights of disabled persons the broader community is becoming increasingly attuned to the notion that handicapped persons should enjoy the same or broadly similar rights as non-handicapped persons (Herr, 1980). This awareness has been heightened by the growth of self-advocacy movements in most western countries. As noted earlier, many parents who have been accustomed to thinking of their handicapped offspring as *eternal children* with circumscribed rights will experience difficulty in accepting the modern view of handicapped persons having rights, especially when such rights are exercised in a way which they perceive to be in conflict with their own interests or those of their handicapped family member.

d) <u>Ensuring satisfactory future provisions for the handicapped person.</u> Of particular concern is what happens to the handicapped person after the incapacitation or death of the parents (Seligman, 1979; 1983). This involves consideration of social as well as economic support for the handicapped person, issues that have been considered in some detail in various guardianship proposals that have been advanced (McLaughlin, 1979; New Zealand Institute of Mental Retardation, 1982). Planning for the future affects siblings as well as parents and for the former is all too frequently surrounded with doubts and ambiguities that can be a major source of anxiety (Skrtic et al., 1983). To help them cope with this task, families need clear information from relevant human service agencies, as well as opportunities to discuss the issues with well-informed professionals (Mittler & Mittler, 1982).

e) <u>Helping the handicapped person gain access to and fulfillment in work and recreational settings.</u> The notion of handicapped persons, particularly those who are mentally handicapped, being considered capable of developing work and

147

recreational skills is relatively new even for *sheltered*
settings (O'Connor & Tizard, 1951), let alone for integrated
settings within the community at large (Bayer & Brown,
1982). As well as demanding well-designed and competently-
staffed rehabilitation, meeting the vocational and leisure
needs of handicapped persons requires a major adjustment on
the part of the broader community (Beck-Ford & Brown, 1984;
Day & Marlett, 1984). This frequently requires, in turn, a
high degree of advocacy on behalf of such persons and their
families.

In the case of the non-handicapped siblings, additional
developmental tasks occur during this stage; these include:

f) Coming to terms with their feelings upon leaving
their family of origin. In some cases, siblings can have
strong feelings of guilt when they leave their parents with
the prime responsibility for caring for the handicapped
person. In others, there is a sense of relief at being able
to pursue their own lives, while in others close relationships are maintained with their handicapped sibling.
Counselling opportunities for siblings should be provided by
service agencies with a view to providing them with assistance in coming to terms with their feelings towards the
handicapped person and their parents. On the whole,
however, there is evidence that only a small majority of
adult siblings felt that having a mentally handicapped
sibling affected commitments in career, marriage and family
(Cleveland & Miller, 1977).

g) Coping with any anxieties regarding their capacity
to be a parent. Siblings of handicapped persons can
identify with them to the extent that they lack confidence
to marry and have children of their own (Simeonsson &
McHale, 1981). In order to counteract any misplaced fears
in this area, as Parfit (1975) has noted, non-handicapped
adolescents need information on the genetic implications of
their sibling's handicap for their own potential offspring.

CONCLUSION

In this chapter, it was argued that the planning, management
and evaluation of services for handicapped persons should be
based on a developmental systems approach. From the systems
perspective, each family should be viewed as comprising a
unique microsystem with complex reciprocal relationships
existing among the family members. Families, in turn, are
embedded in a range of social systems, some of which impinge
very directly on a handicapped person and his or her parents
and siblings, while some have more indirect influences. The

developmental approach leads us to look at the changing patterns and needs of families over the life cycle of the handicapped person.

The following specific principles should form the basis of service planning:

1. The uniqueness of each family microsystem and its interactions with its social environment should be recognized.
2. Since siblings play an important role in families, their contributions should be recognized and their needs met.
3. Given that family structures and needs change over the life cycle of the handicapped person, these should be regularly re-evaluated.
4. Agencies concerned with the health, education and welfare of handicapped persons should be integrated into a whole human service system, centred on the principle of working in partnership with families.
5. Dealing with the broader community's perceptions of handicap and acting as an advocate of handicapped persons is as much the responsibility of professionals as working with a handicapped individual.
6. Successful integration of handicapped persons requires that they and the community be helped to adapt to each other. For the former, this means teaching them social skills and for the latter there should be widespread education on the characteristics and needs of handicapped persons. For both, there must be opportunities to make contact.

REFERENCES

Ackoff, R. & Emery, F. E. (1972) *On Purposeful Systems,* Tavistock Publications, London.

Alpert, J. L. (1981) 'Theoretical Perspectives on the Family Life Cycle,' *The Counselling Psychologist, 9,* 25-33.

Annison, J. E. & Young, W. H. L. (1980) 'The Future Forms of Residential Services for Mentally Retarded People in Australia - A Delphi Study,' *Australian Journal of Developmental Disabilities, 6,* 167-180.

Bayer, M. B. & Brown, R. I. (1982) *Benefits and Costs of Rehabilitation at the Vocational and Rehabilitation Research Institute,* Health and Welfare, Canada.

Bayley, M. (1973) *Mental Handicap and Community Care,* Routledge and Kegan Paul, London.

Beck-Ford, V. & Brown, R. I. (1984) *Leisure Training and Rehabilitation: A Program Manual,* Charles C. Thomas, Springfield, Illinois.

Bell, R. Q. & Harper, L. V. (1977) (eds.) *Child Effects on Adults*, Lawrence Erlbaum, Hillsdale, New Jersey.

Brazelton, T. B., Koslowski, B. & Main, M. (1974) 'The Origins of Reciprocity: The Early Mother-Infant Interaction,' in M. Lewis and L. A. Rosenblum (eds.), *The Effect of the Infant on Its Caregiver*, John Wiley, New York.

Bristol, M. M. & Gallagher, J. J. (1982) 'A Family Focus for Intervention,' in C. Ramey and P. Trohanis (eds.), *Finding and Educating the High Risk and Handicapped Infant*, University Park Press, Baltimore.

Broderick, D. & Smith, J. (1979) 'The General Systems Approach to the Family,' in W. R. Burr, R. Hill, F. I. Nye and I. L. Reiss (eds.), *Contemporary Theories About the Family*, Vol. II, The Free Press, New York.

Bronfenbrenner, U. (1979) *The Ecology of Human Development*, Harvard University Press, Cambridge, Massachusetts.

Bromwich, R. M. (1981) *Working with Parents*, University Park Press, Baltimore.

Brown, R. I. & Hughson, E. A. (1980) *Training of the Developmentally Handicapped Adult*, C. C. Thomas, Springfield, Illinois.

Bruininks, R. H., Thurlow, M. L., Thurman, S. K. & Fiorelli, J. S. (1980) 'Deinstitutionalization and Community Services,' *Mental Retardation and Developmental Disabilities*, 11, 55-101.

Burr, W. R. (1973) *Theory Construction and the Sociology of the Family*, John Wiley and Sons, New York.

Carr, J. (1975) *Young Children with Down's Syndrome*, Butterworths, London.

Challela, M. L. (1981) 'Helping Parents Cope with a Profoundly Mentally Retarded Child,' in A. Milunsky (ed.), *Coping with Crisis and Handicap*, Plenum Press, New York.

Clarke-Stewart, K. A. (1978) 'And Daddy Makes Three: The Father's Impact on Mother and Young Child, *Child Development*, 49, 466-478.

Cleveland, D. W. & Miller, N. (1977) 'Attitudes and Life Commitments of Older Siblings of Mentally Retarded Adults: An Exploratory Study,' *Mental Retardation*, 15, 38-41.

Cunningham, C. C. & Sloper, T. (1977) 'Parents of Down's Syndrome Babies: Their Early Needs,' *Child Care Health and Development*, 3, 325-347.

Day, H. & Marlett, N. (1984) 'Vocational Rehabilitation and Employment,' in N. J. Marlett, R. Gall, and A. Wight-Felske (eds.), *Dialogue on Disability: A Canadian Perspective*, University of Calgary Press, Calgary.

Duff, R. & Campbell, A. (1973) 'Moral and Ethical Dilemmas in the Special Care Nursery,' *New England Journal of Medicine*, 289, 890-894.

Dunlap, W. R. & Hollingsworth, J. S. (1977) 'How Does a Handicapped Child Affect the Family? Implications for Practitioners,' *Family Coordinator, 26,* 286-293.

Farber, B. (1962) 'Effects of a Severely Mentally Retarded Child on the Family,' in E. P. Trapp and P. Himmelstein (eds.), *Readings on the Exceptional Child,* Appleton Century-Crofts, New York.

Featherstone, H. (1981) *A Difference in the Family: Living with a Disabled Child,* Penguin Books, Harmondsworth.

Feiring, C. & Lewis, M. (1978) 'The Child as a Member of the Family System,' *Behavioral Science, 23,* 225-233.

Field, T. M. (1979) 'Interaction Patterns of Preterm and Term Infants,' in T. M. Field, A. Sostek, S. Goldberg and H. Shuman (eds.), *Infants Born at Risk: Behavior and Development,* SP Medical and Scientific Books, New York.

Field, T. M., Widmayer, S. M., Stringer, S. & Ignatoff, E. (1980) 'Teenage Lower-Class Black Mothers and Their Preterm Infants: An Intervention and Developmental Follow-Up,' *Child Development, 51,* 426-436.

Friedrich, W. N. (1979) 'Predictors of the Coping Behaviour of Mothers of Handicapped Children,' *Journal of Consulting and Clinical Psychology, 47,* 1140-1141.

Friedrich, W. N. & Friedrich, W. L. (1981) 'Psychological Assets of Parents of Handicapped and Nonhandicapped Children,' *American Journal of Mental Deficiency, 85,* 551-553.

Gallagher, J. J., Cross, A. & Scharfman, W. (1981) 'Parental Adaptation to a Young Handicapped Child: The Father's Role,' *Journal of the Division for Early Childhood, 3,* 3-14.

Gayton, W. F. (1975) 'Management Problems of Mentally Retarded Children and Their Families,' *Pediatric Clinics of North America, 22,* 561-570.

Gayton, W. F. & Walker, L. (1974) 'Down's Syndrome: Informing the Parents,' *American Journal of Disorders of Childhood, 127,* 510-512.

German, M. L. & Maisto, A. A. (1982) 'The Relationship of a Perceived Family Support System to the Institutional Placement of Mentally Retarded Children,' *Education and Training of the Mentally Retarded, 17,* 17-23.

Griffiths, D. E. (1964) 'The Nature and Meaning of Theory,' in D. E. Griffiths (ed.), *Behavioral Science and Educational Administration,* National Society for the Study of Education, University of Chicago Press, Chicago.

Grossman, F. K. (1972) *Brothers and Sisters of Retarded Children,* Syracuse University Press, Syracuse.

Guess, D., Dussault, B., Brown, F., Mulligan, M., Orelove, F., Comegys, A., & Rues, J. (1984) *Legal, Economic, Psychological and Moral Considerations on the Practice of Withholding Medical Treatment from Infants With Congenital Defects,* Monograph No. 1, The Association for Persons with Severe Handicaps, Seattle.

Hardman, M. L. (1984) 'The Role of Congress in Decisions Relating to the Withholding of Medical Treatment from Seriously Ill Newborns,' *TASH Journal, 9,* 3-7.

Hare, van C. (1967) *Systems Analysis: A Diagnostic Approach,* Harcourt Brace and World, New York.

Havighurst, R. J. (1972) *Developmental Tasks and Education,* 3rd edition, David McKay, New York.

Herr, S. S. (1980) 'Rights of Disabled Persons: International Principles and American Experiences,' *Columbia Human Rights Law Review, 12,* 1-55.

Hewett, S. (1970) *The Family and the Handicapped Child,* Allen and Unwin, London.

Hill, R. (1949) *Families Under Stress,* Harper and Row, New York.

Hornby, G. (in press) 'Families with Exceptional Children,' in D. R. Mitchell and N. N. Singh (eds.), *Exceptional Children in New Zealand,* Dunmore Press, Palmerston North, New Zealand.

Howard, J. (1978) 'The Influence of Children's Developmental Dysfunctions in Marital Quality and Family Interaction,' in R. M. Lerner and G. B. Spanier (eds.), *Child Influences on Marital and Family Interaction,* Academic Press, New York.

Johnson, P. R. (1984) 'Interpersonal Relationships: Self Esteem, Sexual Intimacy and Life-Long Learning,' in R. I. Brown (ed.), *Integrated Programmes for Handicapped Adolescents and Adults,* Croom Helm, London.

Katz, L. G. (1980) 'Mothering and Teaching - Some Significant Distinctions,' in L. G. Katz (ed.), *Current Topics in Early Childhood Education,* Vol. III, Ablex.

Kew, S. (1975) *Handicap and Family Crisis: A Study of Siblings of Handicapped Children,* Pitman, London.

Lamb, M. E. (1983) 'Fathers of Exceptional Children,' in M. Seligman (ed.), *The Family with a Handicapped Child,* Grune and Stratton, New York.

Lewis, M. & Feiring, C. (1980) 'Some American Families at Dinner,' in L. Laosa and I. Sigel (eds.), *The Family as a Learning Environment,* Vol 1, Plenum, New York.

Lipton, H. L. & Svarstad, B. (1977) 'Sources of Variation in Clinicians' Communication to Parents about Mental Retardation,' *American Journal of Mental Deficiency, 82,* 155-161.

Lonsdale, C. (1978) 'Family Life with a Handicapped Child: The Parents Speak,' *Child Care, Health and Development, 4,* 99-120.

Lytton, H. (1980) *Parent-Child Interaction*, Plenum Press, New York.

McConachie, H. (1982) 'Fathers of Mentally Handicapped Children,' in N. Beail and J. McGuire (eds.), *Psychological Aspects of Fatherhood*, Junction, London.

McCubbin, H. I., Joy, C. B., Cauble, A. E., Cameau, J. K., Patterson, J. M. & Needle, R. H. (1980) 'Family Stress and Coping: A Decade Review,' *Journal of Marriage and the Family, 42*, 855-871.

McLaughlin, P. (1979) *Guardianship of the Person*, National Institute on Mental Retardation, Downsview, Ontario.

Meyerson, R. C. (1983) 'Family and Parent Group Therapy,' in M. Seligman (ed.), *The Family with a Handicapped Child: Understanding and Treatment*, Grune and Stratton, New York.

Miller, J. G. (1978) *Living Systems*, McGraw-Hill, New York.

Minuchin, S. (1974) *Families and Family Therapy*, Harvard University Press, Cambridge, Massachusetts.

Mitchell, D. R. (1978) 'A Systems Approach to Designing and Evaluating Special Education,' in A. H. Fink (ed.), *International Perspectives on Future Special Education*, The Council for Exceptional Children, Reston, Virginia.

Mitchell, D. R. (1981a) 'A Survey of Parents' Experiences and Views on Being Told They Have a Handicapped Child,' *New Zealand Medical Journal, 94*, 263-265.

Mitchell, D. R. (1981b) *Other People Don't Really Understand: A Survey of Parents of Young Children with Special Needs*, Project PATH, University of Waikato, Hamilton.

Mitchell, D. R. (ed.) (1982) *Your Child is Different*, George Allen and Unwin, Sydney.

Mitchell, D. R. (1983a) 'Helping Parents to Help Parents: A Workshop on Mutual Support Counselling for Parents of Persons with Handicaps,' Paper presented at a conference on Communication and Children with Special Needs, Wellington, New Zealand.

Mitchell, D. R. (1983b) 'International Trends in Special Education,' *The Canadian Journal of Mental Retardation, 33*, 6-13.

Mitchell, D. R. (1984) 'The Family as Partner - The Parents and Siblings,' Paper presented at the Third Pacific Regional Conference of the International League of Societies for the Mentally Handicapped, Wellington, New Zealand.

Mitchell, D. R. (1985) 'Guidance Needs and Counselling of Parents of Mentally Retarded Persons,' in N. N. Singh and K. M. Wilton (eds.), *Mental Retardation: Research and Services in New Zealand*, Whitcoulls, Christchurch.

Mittler, P. (1984) 'Quality of Life and Services for People with Disabilities,' *Bulletin of The British Psychological Society, 37*, 218-225.

Mittler, P. & McConachie, H. (eds.) (1983) *Parents, Professionals and Mentally Handicapped People: Approaches to Partnership,* Croom Helm, London.

Mittler, P. & Mittler, H. (1982) 'Partnership with Parents,' Stratford-upon-Avon, National Council for Special Education.

New Zealand Institute of Mental Retardation (1982) *Guardianship for Mentally Retarded Adults: Submissions to the Minister of Justice,* New Zealand Institute of Mental Retardation, Wellington.

Nock, S. L. (1982) 'The Life Cycle Approach to Family Analysis,' in B. Wolman (ed.), *Handbook of Developmental Psychology,* Prentice Hall, Englewood Cliffs.

O'Connor, N. & Tizard, J. (1951) 'Predicting the Occupational Adequacy of Certified Mental Defectives,' *Occupational Psychology, 25,* 205-211.

O'Hara, D. M., Chaiklin, H. & Mosher, B. S. (1980) 'A Family Life Cycle Plan for Delivering Services to the Developmentally Handicapped,' *Child Welfare, 59,* 80-90.

Parfit, J. (1975) 'Siblings of Handicapped Children,' *Special Education: Forward Trends, 2,* 19-21.

Parke, R. D. (1978) 'Parent-Infant Interaction: Progress, Paradigms and Problems,' in G. P. Sackett (ed.), *Observing behavior: Vol. 1, Theory and Applications in Mental Retardation,* University Park Press, Baltimore.

Parke, R. D. & Lewis, N. G. (1981) 'The Family in Context: A Multilevel Interactional Analysis of Child Abuse,' in R. W. Henderson (ed.), *Parent-Child Interaction: Theory, Research and Prospects,* Academic Press, New York.

Pratt, D. (1982) 'A Cybernetic Model for Curriculum Development,' *Instructional Science, 11,* 1-12.

President's Commission for the Study of Ethical Problems in Medicine and Biomedical and Behavioural Research (1983) 'Seriously Ill Newborns,' in *Deciding to Forego Life-sustaining Treatment,* U.S. Government Printing Office, Washington, D.C.

Price-Bonham, S. & Addison, S. (1978) 'Families and Mentally Retarded Children: Emphasis on the Father,' *The Family Coordinator, 27*(1), 221-230.

Pruchno, R. A., Blow, F. O., & Smyer, M. A. (1984) 'Life Events and Interdependent Lives: Implications for Research and Intervention,' *Human Development, 27,* 31-41.

Ramey, C. T., McPhee, D., & Yates, K. D. (1982) 'Preventing Developmental Retardation: A General Systems Model,' in L. Bond and J. Jaffe (eds), *Facilitating Infant and Early Childhood Development,* University Press of New England, Hanover, New Hampshire.

Raye, J. R. & Healey, J. M. (1984) 'The Neonatal Intensive-care Unit: Developing an Acceptable Public Policy,' *Topics in Early Childhood Special Education, 4,* 71-82.

Reiss, D. (1981) *The Family's Construction of Reality,* Harvard University Press, Cambridge, Massachusetts.

Rubin, S. & Quinn-Curran, N. (1983) 'Lost, Then Found: Parents' Journey Through the Community Service Maze,' in M. Seligman (ed.), *The Family with a Handicapped Child: Understanding and Treatment,* Grune and Stratton, New York.

Sanson-Fisher, R. & Maguire, P. (1980) 'Should Skills in Communicating with Patients be Taught in Medical Schools?' *The Lancet,* September 6, 523-526.

Seligman, M. (1979) *Strategies for Helping Parents of Exceptional Children,* The Free Press, New York.

Seligman, M. (1983) *The Family with a Handicapped Child: Understanding and Treatment,* Grune and Stratton, New York.

Shearer, D. (1985) 'Everybody's Ethics: What Future for Handicapped Babies?' *Early Child Development and Care, 18,* 189-216.

Simeonsson, R. J. & McHale, S. (1981) 'Review, Research on Handicapped Children: Sibling Relationships,' *Child Care and Health and Development, 7.*

Simeonsson, R. J. & Simeonsson, N. E. (1981) 'Parenting Handicapped Children: Psychological Aspects,' in J. L. Paul (ed), *Understanding and Working with Parents of Children with Special Needs,* Holt, Rinehart and Winston, New York.

Skrtic, T. M., Summers, J. A., Brotherson, M. J., & Turnbull, A. P. (1983) 'Severely Handicapped Children and their Brothers and Sisters,' in J. Blacher (ed.), *Young Severely Handicapped Children and their Families: Research in Review,* Academic Press, New York.

Spain, B. & Wigley, G. (1975) *Right from the Start,* National Society for Mentally Handicapped Children, London.

Stewart, N. R., Winborn, B. B., Johnson, R. G., Burks, H. M., & Engelkes, J. R. (eds.) (1978) *Systematic Counseling,* Prentice Hall, Englewood Cliffs.

Strickland, B. (1983) 'Legal Issues that Affect Parents,' in M. Seligman (ed.), *The Family with a Handicapped Child: Understanding and Treatment,* Grune and Stratton, New York.

Suelzle, M. & Keenan, V. (1981) 'Changes in Family Support Networks Over the Life Cycle of Mentally Retarded Persons,' *American Journal of Mental Deficiency, 86,* 267-274.

Todres, D., Krane, D., Howell, M. C. & Shannon, D. C. (1977) 'Pediatricians' Attitudes Affecting Decision-making in Defective Newborns,' *Pediatrics, 60,* 197-201.

Trevino, F. (1979) 'Siblings of Handicapped Children: Identifying Those at Risk,' *The Journal of Contemporary Social Work, 60,* 488-492.

Turnbull, A. P., Brotherson, M. J. & Summers, J. A. (1983) 'The Impact of Deinstitutionalization on Families: A Family Systems Approach,' in R. H. Bruininks (ed.), *Living and Learning in the Least Restrictive Environment,* Paul H. Brookes Publishing Co., Baltimore.

Von Bertalanffy, L. (1968) *General Systems Theory,* George Braziller, New York.

Wikler, L. (1981) 'Chronic Stresses of Families of Mentally Retarded Children. Family Relations,' *Journal of Applied Family and Child Studies, 30,* 2.

Wikler, L., Wasow, M. & Hatfield, E. (1981) 'Chronic Sorrow Revisited: Parent vs Professional Depiction of the Adjustment of Parents of Mentally Retarded Children,' *American Journal of Orthopsychiatry, 51,* 63-70.

Wilkin, D. (1979) *Caring for the Mentally Handicapped Child,* Croom Helm, London.

Wing, L. (1975) 'Problems Experienced by Parents of Children with Severe Mental Retardation,' in B. Spain and G. Wigley (eds), *Right from the Start,* National Society for Mentally Handicapped Children, London.

Wolraich, M. L. & Reiter, S. (1979) 'Training Physicians in Communication Skills,' *Developmental Medicine and Child Neurology, 21,* 773-778.

Chapter Eight

VOCATIONAL REHABILITATION SYSTEMS AND STRUCTURES: A
BI-NATIONAL LOOK

Shunit Reiter, Diane N. Bryen, Edward Newman and
Yecheskel Taler

INTRODUCTION

The purpose of this chapter is to describe two contrasting
organizational systems and structures in vocational
rehabilitation settings in Israel and in the United States.
The implications of these two systems on programmes,
personnel, and clients will be discussed.

A common outlook exists in the two countries on a
conceptual definition, criteria of client success, and
stages of the rehabilitation process. However, subtle yet
important differences between the two countries also exist
in the rehabilitation systems and the organizational and
management styles which affect programme orientation,
personnel, and clients.

American and Israeli vocational rehabilitation leaders
appear to be comfortable with the definition proposed by the
National Council of Rehabilitation (New York, 1942)
according to which *Rehabilitation is the dynamic process in
which a disabled person is helped to discover, fulfill and
develop his physical, emotional, mental, social and
occupational potentials to their utmost* (Katz and Florian,
1975).

A second shared aspect of the two rehabilitation
systems relates to *criteria for clients' success.* The
attainment of work and economic independence are seen in
both countries as major goals of rehabilitation and as
significant criteria for measuring the success of the
rehabilitation process.

The third area in which there is a shared view among
American and Israeli rehabilitation leaders is in the *stages
of the rehabilitation process.* It is generally accepted
that a comprehensive programme should include (Katz &
Florian, 1975; Bolton, 1976):

1) outreach and screening of the population to be served,
2) comprehensive individual assessment,
3) counselling,
4) developing and implementing training programmes,
5) the provision of other needed services,
6) placement in the community,
7) follow up.

The notion that the rehabilitation process is not unidirectional is accepted by both countries. If a client is not showing progress at a particular stage of the rehabilitation process, he may return to any previous stage.

Thus, despite the many socio-cultural differences between the United States and Israel (Bryen, Reiter, & Newman, 1985), in the area of rehabilitation there is general agreement with the conceptual definition of rehabilitation, general criteria for measuring client success, and the stages of the rehabilitation process. Major differences between the two countries lie mainly in the organization of the rehabilitation system in general, and in the operation of the rehabilitation facilities in particular, which may be themselves reflections of the two different social orders.

Not much research has been carried out on the relationship between the organization and structure of rehabilitation services and client outcome. This might be due to the fact that when the rehabilitation service is evaluated the focus is either on the professional staff or on the general and local economic situation. This, as described by Lorenz (1983), is usually the case when researchers and policy makers ask the question *why don't we have more placements rather than less?*

We frequently hear that the problem is the economy - there are not enough jobs available - or that the problem is that counsellors do not know how to place clients. These variables, while important, are not the only variables that should be investigated. The organization and structure of the rehabilitation system is no less crucial for the success of the service.

Vocational rehabilitation services are provided within human service organizations which may lack a clear concept of organizational effectiveness, more specifically, a consensus as to what constitutes successful client outcomes. According to Imershein, Chackerian, Martin and Frumkin (1983), this uncertainty has been typically dealt with by a heavy reliance on the skills and judgment of its professionals. Thus, rehabilitation counsellors, workshop supervisors, social workers, physicians, nurses, psychologists, special educators and others involved in rehabilitation services, are an important factor in defining the content areas of rehabilitation, its scope, and its criteria for success. These individual professionals, on the one hand, are the ones who define the services given to clients, while on the other hand service effectiveness is also dependent upon how well their efforts are coordinated and organized by the human service organizations carrying out these rehabilitation services. Furthermore the human service organizations are influenced by the political and economic environment.

The formal structure of the organization of the rehabilitation system is not always determined by demands emanating from assessed client needs or from current rehabilitation practices, but by policy makers who are generally removed from these needs and practices. Although we find general agreement in Israel and in America on conceptual definitions of rehabilitation and its goals and stages, organizations serving handicapped persons and their inter-organizational relationships are structured differently. It is, therefore, useful to describe the organizational structures in both countries to understand better the relationships between the structure, the rehabilitation process, and client outcome.

In this chapter we will follow the classification suggested by Imershein, Chackerian, Martin and Frumkin (1983) using the four sets of variables to be considered in rehabilitation research of this nature:

1. Demands and controls exercised by the political components of the organization's environment,
2. The organization's structure,
3. The delivery of services by the organization,
4. Clients' demands for and responses to service.

The focus of the chapter will be on facilities characterized as vocational rehabilitation centres. Two centres will be described, one in Israel the other in America, with special emphasis on their political environments, their internal structure, the services they offer clients and the possible impact on clients.

ISRAEL

The Vocational Rehabilitation System

In Israel, a nation of approximately four million persons, there is a general absence of coherent, formalized, and legislatively-backed national or sub-national plans and philosophies of rehabilitation. This absence reinforces diversity in both the philosophy and modes of service delivery. Goals and philosophies range through preventive

159

to rehabilitative to maintenance, with service delivery modes ranging from *end point* placement in vocational workshops to competitive employment. Basic laws in the area of social services were enacted in the first decades after the establishment of the State. The laws bring together the pre-state provisions at a general level. Agencies operating under the general authority of basic laws have considerable discretion regarding the development of programmes which, in turn, frequently reflect the predilections of programme heads in concert with interest and consumer groups.

Principal basic laws include those concerning compulsory education (1949), a State education system (1953), national insurance (1954), care for persons with mental illness (1955), social welfare (1958), employment service (1959), and general disability (1974). In the absence of legislatively-formalized national plans, programmes and services for persons with disabilities are often established and managed by strong-willed and determined individuals who conceive and develop a local rehabilitation programme, hire and lead staff, establish personalized relationships with clients, and remain in leadership or *boss* roles over a period of years.

There are a number of national agencies that deal directly with the vocational rehabilitation of handicapped persons. They are: the *National Insurance Institute, Division of Rehabilitation*; the *Ministry of Labour and Social Affairs*, including the *Department of Rehabilitation* and its *Fund for Rehabilitation Centres*; the *Ministry of Defense, Department of Rehabilitation*; and *Hameshakem Ltd.* (in English: the rehabilitator). These agencies cover most of the vocational rehabilitation services in the country. Few non-governmental organizations are involved in the delivery of vocational rehabilitation services without substantial public support. All of the above agencies share the common goal of assisting disabled individuals, such as elderly persons, people with physical disabilities, those with mental handicaps, emotional illness and those experiencing cultural and social disadvantage, to develop their work potential to the utmost and, following training, find work in sheltered or open employment.

The National Insurance Institute (NII) provides social security payments to special groups in the population. In 1982, over 67,000 persons were on the disabilities roles for reasons other than war. It has been its policy since 1954 to assist handicapped people in obtaining vocational rehabilitation services. Thus, such persons are being trained or re-trained for remunerative employment. The NII attempts through community outreach programmes to locate all eligible people who may be unaware of their rights to rehabilitation services. It also provides comprehensive social, vocational and medical assessment of the individual; development of individual rehabilitation plans and referral to other agencies which might assist the individual according to the NII's plan.

The Division of Rehabilitation is NII's administrative and professional arm for vocational rehabilitation. The Division is composed of 165 rehabilitation officers, most of them social workers. It is at the headquarters that policy is defined and decided upon. There, client data from all over the country are nationally registered and assessment, case planning and treatment are initiated and implemented.

The Rehabilitation Department of the Ministry of Labour and Social Affairs is the largest agency in Israel responsible for the vocational rehabilitation of all disabled, handicapped and socially and economically disadvantaged persons from birth to age 65 living in the community. Its services include:

- social, vocational, psychological and medical
  evaluations of clients;
- vocational guidance and counselling;
- psychological, social and medical treatment;
- pre-vocational programmes;
- selective placements in sheltered or open employment;
- and follow up of clients.

The Department operates several vocational rehabilitation centres mainly through the Fund for Rehabilitation Centres.

The Fund was created in 1965 with the specific purpose of developing and operating vocational rehabilitation centres and sheltered workshops for the disabled. The Fund has two separate headquarter units, one in Jerusalem at the Ministry of Labour and Social Affairs, mainly responsible for policy and professional supervision, the other in Tel Aviv at the administrative headquarters of the Fund, responsible for the running of rehabilitation centres. The Fund operates 15 vocational rehabilitation centres, six sheltered workshops, two vocational training centres for school drop outs as well as providing occupations for home bound people. The centre to be described in this chapter is one of those operated by the Fund.

Hameshakem, Ltd. began its operation in 1962 as a joint agency between the Ministry of Labour and Social Affairs and the Jewish Agency. Its initial purpose was that of finding and providing employment for new immigrants. Since then it has expanded its population to include elderly and disabled persons. It operates mainly through sheltered workshops. Its board of directors includes four Government and two Jewish Agency representatives.

Ministry of Defense, Department of Rehabilitation began its services in 1948 and serves veterans with physical, sensory, and emotional handicaps, and veterans who are brain damaged or who have social handicaps (the latter must be combined with a physical or mental handicap). Its services include: diagnosis, development of individualized service plans, job placement, and follow-up after placement. Outcome criteria include how well the individual functions at work, within his or her family, and in society. A disabled person may be served by this agency throughout his or her lifetime. Sixty thousand families receive some type of service each month.

From an analysis of the policies and organization of the above agencies, (from the report of the committee that investigated the coordination of the rehabilitation services in Israel, 1984), it appears that organizations provide similar services to similar handicapped populations, often with similar goals. In addition, the concentrated efforts of these agencies are not well coordinated. The result of this is the relative isolation of each agency. Thus, although a large proportion of clients in each particular rehabilitation centre has been referred from different agencies, i.e. the NII, the Defense Ministry, or the Labour and Welfare Ministry, each local centre is relatively independent of the policies of the referring agency. Each centre is funded by its own agency but is not accountable to the referring agencies. Moreover, there is no one main, central body where the different agencies dealing with rehabilitation work together to coordinate their efforts. Thus, on the national level, (similar in size and scope to a state in the United States) each agency works in relative isolation from the others.

Figure 1 illustrates the referral process from each particular agency to the particular rehabilitation centre.

The Organizational Structure of the Centre

For the purposes of this chapter a vocational rehabilitation centre was chosen as prototypical of the centres operated by the Fund for Rehabilitation Centres. The centre to be described is located in the northern part of Israel, near the city of Acre. The centre draws from rural and urban populations totalling approximately 200,000 people. In early 1984, the rate of unemployment was 8 per cent. The centre's main business/industrial base includes light industry, technical semi-skilled occupations and services. In 1984, the centre served about 690 clients. Its population included: socially disadvantaged youth still in schools to which the centre provided mainly vocational guidance and counselling; physically handicapped individuals; mentally handicapped persons; those with emotional disturbances; and socially and culturally disadvantaged people who are chronically unemployed. The publicly stated goals of the centre are:

1) the return of clients to the regular work force and the enhancement of normal and acceptable social behavior,
2) developing treatment and rehabilitation methods according to the special needs of the population served,
3) raising community awareness to the work of the centre and its special contributions in the areas of vocational assessment, guidance, and training.

The centre's staff (n=24) include: a director, administrative assistants (a secretary and a telephonist), a workshop coordinator, a social welfare coordinator, an assessment and evaluation coordinator, a youth evaluator, an adult evaluator, a house mother, six workshop supervisors, six social workers, a placement officer, a youth project coordinator, a psychologist, and a continuing education teacher. The staff/client ratio for the 85 clients who are receiving ongoing vocational training is 1 to 8. The employees at the Centre are not highly professionalized (i.e. generally at the baccalaureate level) and a background in social work is the most frequent academic qualification. The social work orientation of the Centre is also reflected in the relatively large number of social workers employed. There is little specialization of staff roles. Several responsibilities (i.e. counselling, training, follow-up) are embedded within an individual staff member's role.

As illustrated in Figure 2, the functional organization of the centre is fairly non-hierarchical. At the head is a director who is directly responsible to the headquarters of the Fund for Rehabilitation centres. Reporting to him are the coordinators of the major services of the centre and they are in charge of the frontline staff. The director of the centre is both the administrative and the professional head. Each member of the staff is equally free to approach the director if he or she has any query, complaint, or special need. The coordinators are mainly responsible for the smooth running of the programmes and will refer personal concerns of staff directly to the director. The director therefore personally knows and deals with all staff members - whether administrative, maintenance, or professional.

FIGURE 1 REFERRAL PROCESS TO COMPETITIVE EMPLOYMENT AND SHELTERED WORK FOR PEOPLE WITH HANDICAPS: ISRAEL

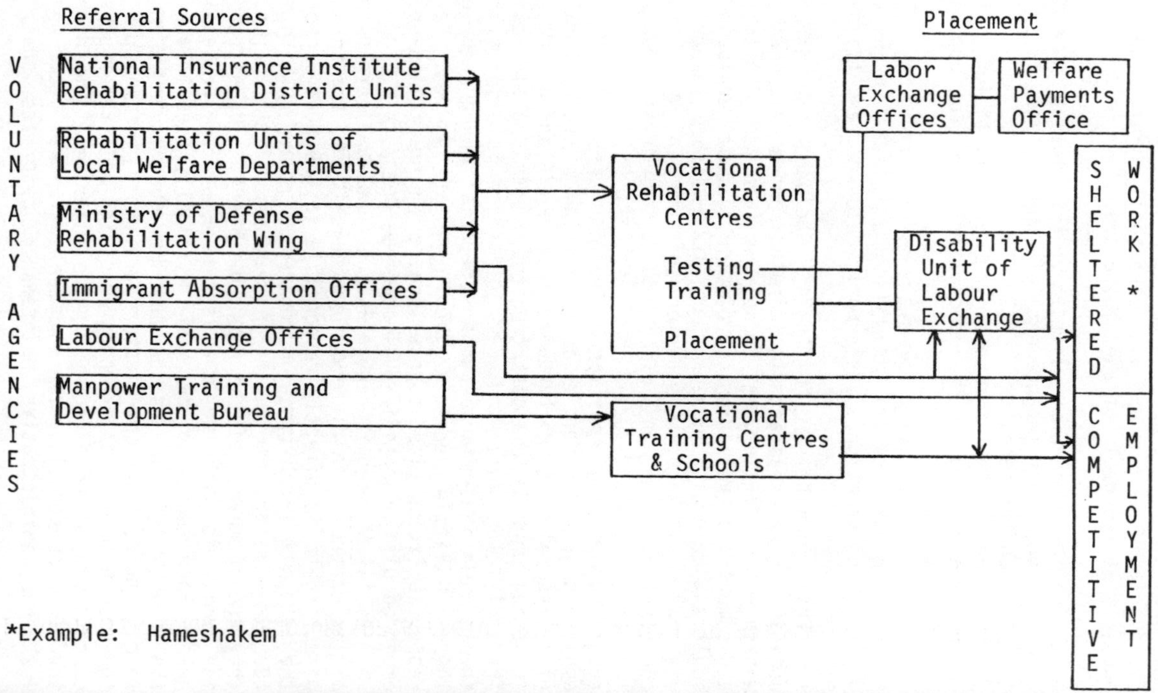

Developmental Systems Approach

164

FIGURE 2 ORGANIZATIONAL STRUCTURE OF A PROTOTYPICAL ISRAELI VOCATIONAL REHABILITATION CENTRE

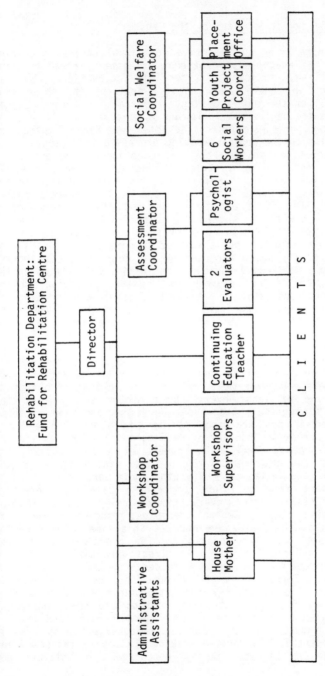

The Delivery of Services by the Centre

The centre is a comprehensive vocational centre, providing vocational education, vocational assessment, rehabilitation counselling, training in specific occupational skills, training in general work habits, training in job seeking skills, on-the-job training, referrals to work places outside the centre and follow up of clients.

For purposes of this chapter we have focused our attention on the decision-making process at the centre. The first decision relates to the acceptance or rejection of clients referred by a variety of agencies (see Figure 1). The social welfare coordinator is the first to receive the file, and, in consultation with one of the centre's social workers, the first evaluation is conducted. The director sees the new client's file but is generally not involved in the initial evaluation of clients unless consulted. If the client is accepted, he is invited to come to the centre. On his first day he is escorted by the centre's social worker who shows him around and gives an initial orientation to the centre. Following comprehensive social, psychological and vocational assessments, a multi-disciplinary meeting is called of all those involved in the specific case: the referring agency, the psychologist, the evaluator, the social worker, the centre's director or the centre's social welfare coordinator, and the client himself. The rehabilitation programme for the client is then devised taking into account as much as possible the client's wishes and ideas. Regular meetings are then held at each turning point and at least every three months to evaluate the client's progress. Subsequent decisions are made by those involved in his training, mainly his supervisor and his social worker (counsellor or case manager). Towards the end of the process other professionals might be involved, for example the placement officer, the continuing education teacher, and in the case of youth, their parents.

Apart from decisions concerning clients, there are general staff meetings every Friday morning when no training is taking place. General decisions concerning the programmes at the centre are made at this time. The director is present at these meetings. The coordinators of programmes and staff involved in direct work with clients are also present and involved in the decision-making process.

To a large extent the director of the centre and his staff form a relatively autonomous unit and have a fair amount of freedom to try new methods and new programmes. The director, though he follows general rules and regulations issued by the Fund's headquarters, is fairly independent in his decision-making ability to try new ideas and new techniques. He is encouraged to initiate new projects and even to apply for funding to agencies other than the Fund.

The director of the centre sets the tone as far as formal and informal relations are concerned. Since there are no written and formal job descriptions of positions, staff are generally free to create their job according to their and the director's understanding of the centre's basic goals and methods. The director may grant reasonable independence to the staff in their interpretation of their work. Paper work is limited to general descriptions of client's individual programme plans and the decisions made at the multidisciplinary meetings.

Client's Demands for and Responses to Service

The attitude of the director and the staff is that their main accountability is towards individual clients *and* their families and, only to a lesser extent, towards the Fund and the general community. Clients are therefore encouraged to show initiative and independence. At each turning point in their programme, decisions are thoroughly explained to them. Clients are encouraged to react to decisions, and to express their feelings and attitudes. If negative, staff try to explain and reason with clients, and in some cases, modify programmes. The consent of clients to the programmes devised for them and their willingness to follow the programmes are considered important.

Considering the fact that there are not many levels of professionals and administrators between the individual client and the director, clients have easy access to the director and the coordinators. The director is known to all clients and he also knows, even if superficially, most of them, especially those in long term training programmes.

Clients generally remain at the centre for up to a year. Client outcome is determined by this participatory and interactive process and may include any combination of employment, personal adjustment or skill development objectives.

THE UNITED STATES

The Vocational Rehabilitation System

The most venerable framework for helping handicapped persons in the United States is known as the vocational rehabilitation system. Like Israel, the United States lacks a comprehensive national programme which legislatively or administratively links all programmes into a coordinated network. Those who viewed the rehabilitation system as a comprehensive approach to the whole problem of disability were over-optimistic. However, unlike Israel, Federal legislation has had direct and specific impact on rehabilitation facilities and their programmes and services in the United States.

The federal government spends over $20 billion on disability and disability-related programmes under the Social Security Act, as well as through support for special education and some employment training programmes. The traditional federal-state vocational rehabilitation programme, with a 1984 federal authorization of just over one billion dollars, provides a small proportion of service and benefits in an expanding benefit/service universe. This is reflected in the increasingly diverse funding base used by rehabilitation facilities to provide services and training to individuals all the while having to comply to federal, state and local rules and regulations.

Volumes have been written which describe or *map* the many agencies and programmes subsumed under the label of rehabilitation. Therefore, only a brief description will be provided of those agencies that deal directly with the vocational rehabilitation of persons with handicaps or which indirectly affect vocational rehabilitation outcome.

The Rehabilitation Services Administration (RSA) in the Department of Education administers grants to states, on a fiscally matched basis, for the provision of vocational rehabilitation services for physically and/or mentally disabled individuals. Services provided or funded through state agencies (i.e. Offices of Vocational Rehabilitation) include diagnosis, counselling, vocational training and placement, and physical and mental restoration. To qualify for RSA support for vocational rehabilitation services through a state agency, an individual must have a physical or mental disability which limits him/her from obtaining, retaining, or preparing for employment consistent with the individual's capabilities. Additionally, the state agency must determine that the individual will benefit from rehabilitation services in terms of employability. Each state agency establishes specific procedures for appraising an individual's eligibility. If eligible, state agencies refer individuals to and purchase services from public or private facilities, such as the rehabilitation centre. The costs are met in part by the government. The rehabilitation centres provide or procure physical, medical, and rehabilitation services and attempt to integrate medical, psychological, social and vocational aspects. Vocationally-oriented rehabilitation programmes, of which there are several thousand in operation, use work activity as a method of providing vocational evaluation, work adjustment, and sheltered employment services.

The Social Security Administration (SSA), in the Department of Health and Human Services, pays disability benefits to individuals meeting specific criteria. A disability is defined as the inability to do any substantial gainful activity (e.g. work) because of a medically-determined physical or mental impairment which has lasted or can be expected to last at least 12 months or result in death.

Authorized state agencies, such as the state welfare department, or the SSA when no such agency exists, determine eligibility based on data submitted by the individual. If the individual does not follow prescribed treatments, returns to gainful employment, or is determined to be no longer disabled, benefits are discontinued.

The essential difference between SSA and RSA is that SSA primarily provides payments directly to persons and RSA primarily supports the provision of services through state vocational rehabilitation agencies.

The Veterans Administration (VA) conducts many programmes that provide substantial benefits and services to disabled veterans, including medical and vocational rehabilitation. In some cases a veteran may receive complementary services from both the VA and the state rehabilitation agency.

State Employment Services are part of a national system known as the United States Employment Services (USES) of the Department of Labour. The system is charged with placing persons in employment and serving employers seeking qualified individuals to fill job openings. Every local office is required to designate at least one staff member to help individuals with handicaps receive service and ensures equal opportunity for employment and equal pay commensurate to the individual's abilities.

Employment Standards Administration (ESA), also of the Department of Labour, is involved with handicapped workers subject to the Fair Labour Standards Act who cannot earn at least the minimum wage because of their handicaps. The Act allows for subminimum wage certification when necessary and for the shortest period necessary to prevent curtailment of opportunity for individuals with handicaps. State rehabilitation agencies are authorized by the Department of

Labour to issue temporary subminimum wage exceptions which usually apply to sheltered workshops.

The Office of Selective Placement Programmes of the United States Civil Service Employment implements the federal government's policy of promoting the hiring, placement, and advancement of persons with physical and/or mental handicaps, including disabled veterans. Knowledge and technologies are developed to enhance employment of all groups of people with disabilities. Also technical assistance is provided to federal agencies in the development and implementation of their affirmative action programmes.

The complex vocational rehabilitation system is at the same time *rich* yet uncoordinated. Agencies at the state level have begun to move toward each other to attempt cooperative approaches to the vocational rehabilitation needs of its citizens. Each agency is limited by law (and by funds) to its own mandate, but receives consumer pressures to expand services. The special education agency relinquishes responsibility at young adulthood. The rehabilitation agency can provide only short-term assistance. The employment agency may require special technical assistance as may the agencies for persons with mental retardation or mental disabilities. System change towards increasing competitive and supported employment opportunities will probably begin to unfold at state levels before the federal government develops a coherent and more comprehensive rehabilitation programme and corresponding fiscal policy.

The Organizational Structure of a Prototypical Vocational Rehabilitation Centre

The vocational rehabilitation centre to be described is not atypical of private, nonprofit vocational rehabilitation centres in the United States. It is one centre operated by a large comprehensive vocational and employment agency. The centre is located in a large east coast city, serving suburban and urban populations of approximately 1,700,000. In early 1984, the local unemployment rate was 7.7 per cent. The primary business/industrial base of this area is commerce (wholesale and retail), finance, insurance, real estate, and nonprofessional services. During 1983-1984, the centre served 356 handicapped individuals who suffered from emotional disability, mental handicaps, physical disabilities, visual handicaps, learning disability, and/or social disadvantage. The publicly declared goal of the centre is the vocational rehabilitation of its clients so that they may be successfully employed in the open labour market.

The centre's full-time staff (n=28) include: a director; directors of counselling, physical therapy, training, the business and trades school, and English as a Second Language; manager and assistant manager of the production workshop; assistant director of the business and trade school; clerical office manager and clerical staff; maintenance superintendent and maintenance staff; intake supervisor and counsellors; placement officers; evaluation supervisor, evaluators, and evaluation aides, therapists; foremen, and drivers and handlers; and instructors. The staff/client ratio is one staff member for each 12 clients. The professional staff are more highly trained than in Israel, with academic backgrounds ranging from baccalaureate to doctorates in rehabilitation, psychology, and special education. Not only is there a high degree of professionalization in the centre, but there is also a high degree of specialization of staff roles and functions formalized by written job descriptions.

As illustrated in Figure 3, the organizational structure of the centre is pyramidal and hierarchical in nature. At the top is the director who is directly responsible to the umbrella organization and the various state agencies which fund the centre. In addition, he is responsible for the overall administrative, operational, and fiscal concerns of the centre. Under him are various service directors, and sometimes assistant directors, who are responsible for the specific operations and supervision of staff in their particular service area. Since these are managerial positions, no direct work with clients is provided by these staff members. Line staff, whether instructors, counsellors, therapists, or evaluators, work directly with clients and are directly responsible to their respective directors. As can be seen from this description and from Figure 3, there are several layers of staff separating clients from decision-makers (i.e. the director and service directors). A similar situation exists for direct service staff. As a result, lines of communication are quite formal and generally unidirectional, i.e. from top to bottom. The implications for clients and staff of this organizational structure, especially as it contrasts to the Israeli centre, will be discussed in the final section of this chapter.

Delivery of Services by the Centre

This centre, like the Israeli one, is a comprehensive vocational rehabilitation centre providing vocational evaluation, counselling, work adjustment training, occupational skills training, physical therapy, placement and follow-up on the job.

FIGURE 3   ORGANIZATIONAL STRUCTURE OF A PROTOTYPICAL VOCATIONAL REHABILITATION CENTRE IN THE UNITED STATES

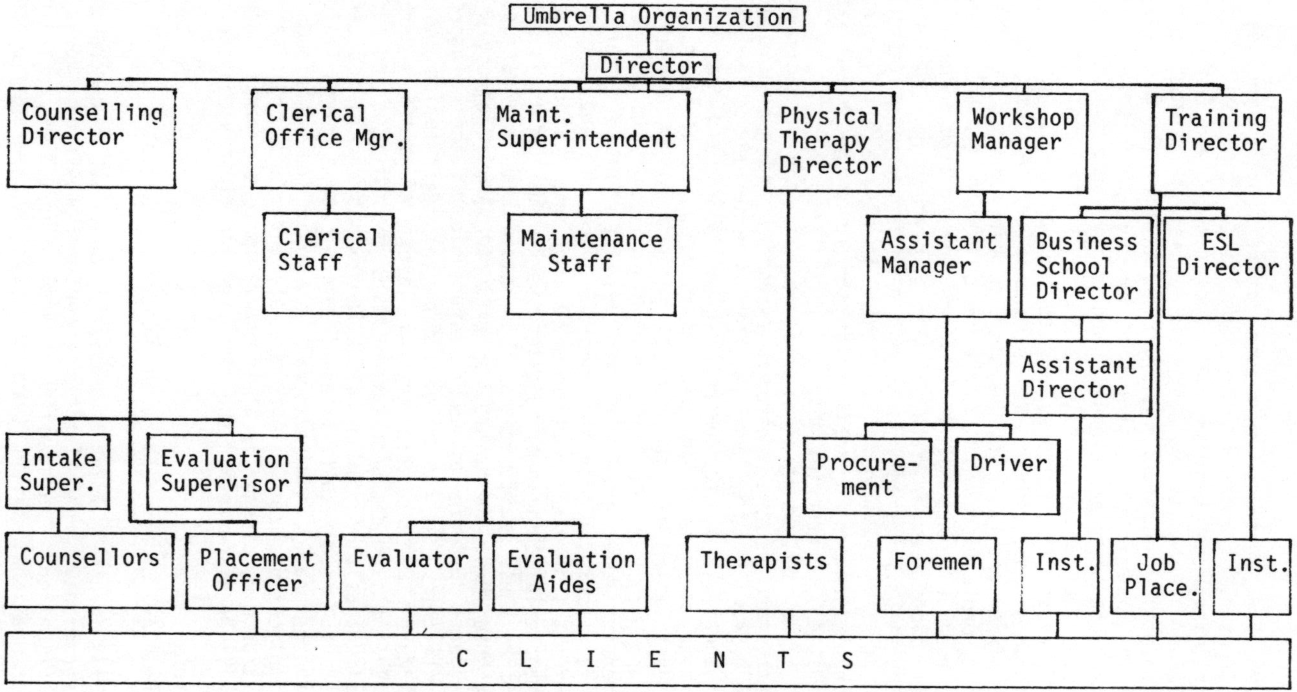

The decision-making process follows formal procedures. Referrals to the centre come from a variety of agencies, including the Office of Vocational Rehabilitation, the Veterans' Administration, Bureau of Blindness, County Office of Mental Health/Mental Retardation, psychiatric hospitals, probation and parole agencies, and private insurance companies. Initial eligibility is determined by these referring agencies and is confirmed by the intake worker at the centre. Eligibility criteria, usually established by the referring, and thus usually the funding, agency includes nature and severity of the handicap and the financial status of the client. Once the centre determines that the client is eligible for vocational services, evaluation begins which lasts, and is funded for, four weeks. During the first two weeks of evaluation, work samples and other vocational tests are administered by the evaluator. This is followed by production evaluation conducted by the foreman and meetings with the case manager to discuss the client's adjustment to the work situation. At the end of the four-week evaluation period, an Individual Work Programme Plan (IWPP) is developed by the case manager, the rehabilitation counsellor, the foreman, and the evaluator. If the client agrees with the proposed IWPP, he/she will provide formal, written consent.

Subsequent decisions relating to the client are made through a formalized mechanism of monthly revised IWPP's, written progress notes each time the client is seen by the counsellor, and through monthly progress reports. When the client demonstrates adequate quality and quantity of work, satisfactory relations with the foreman (authority) and co-workers, satisfactory socialization, attendance, and punctuality as assessed by the foreman and the case manager, the placement officer is brought in and the placement process begins.

While the centre has no strict time limits for vocational rehabilitation, funding constraints from the referring agency (e.g. OVR) do impose very real limits to the duration of vocational training. For example, OVR will fund a client for 20 weeks even though there is a tacit expectation that many clients, because of the severity of their handicaps, will require service for a longer time. As a result, if the centre retains the client it may be at the Centre's own expense. Consequently, after a year if the client has not been placed, he will be either

1) referred to another programme (e.g. a sheltered workshop),
2) strongly encouraged to improve production and work adjustment in order to be placed in competitive employment, or
3) terminated.

Other decisions about or input from the clients occur both formally, through IWPP meetings and grievance procedures, and informally through meetings with their counsellor. Laws and funding considerations have substantial impact on both client rights and staff decisions. As such, staff-client interactions are usually according to precise and formal procedures.

Accountability to funding agencies requires attention to detail and is time-consuming with a great deal of paper work. As much as 50 per cent of a professional staff person's time may be spent providing written documentation of compliance to federal, state, and/or local laws, regulations, and standards.

Client outcome is determined by formalized, yet somewhat subjectively evaluated, sets of criteria (e.g. quality and quantity of production, work habits). Successful employment in the open labour market is the primary outcome to which most programme resources are focused. Other client outcomes, such as skill development and personal adjustment, are subordinated as means to achieving this unitary outcome.

COMPARISONS

Significant similarities and differences exist between the two rehabilitation systems and the two centres described. A comparative summary is provided in Table 1. However, only those differences considered to be significant to the client will be discussed.

TABLE 1   COMPARISONS BETWEEN REHABILITATION CENTRES IN
         ISRAEL AND UNITED STATES

	ISRAEL	UNITED STATES
The Rehabilitation System		
Coherent/comprehensive rehabilitation programme?	No	No
Legislatively-backed services?	No	Some
Referral/point of entry	Few points of entry	Several points of entry

The Rehabilitation Centre	ISRAEL	UNITED STATES
Local population served	200,000 urban & rural	1,700,000 urban & sub-urban
Local unemployment rate (1984)	7.7%	8%
Local business/industry base	light industry; technical & non professional services; agriculture.	Commerce; finance, real estate; non-professional services.
Clients served	ED=36% MR=14% PH=30% Head Injured =15% Other=5%	ED=72% MR=15% PH= 5% Other=8%
Goals of the Centre	Entry into the work force; normal accept-ance & social behaviour.	Employment in the open labour market.

Staff

Staff/client ratio	Approx. 1 to 8	Approx. 1 to 12
Professionalization	Generally BA in social work.	BA through doctoral level in rehabilita-tion, psycho-logy, special education.
Specialization	No formal job descriptions; relative free-dom to create own job based on Centre's goals.	Formal job des-criptions and specialized roles and res-ponsibilities.
Organizational Structure	Flat: lines of communication personal/ informal.	Pyramidal: formal lines of communication.

Delivery of Services by the Centre

	ISRAEL	UNITED STATES
Type of Services	Comprehensive vocational services.	Comprehensive vocational services.
Decisions about client services (nature, duration)	Multidisciplinary; informal - relative autonomy.	Multidisciplinary; formal - influenced by law, rules, and funding agencies.
Accountability	Relative autonomy; limited paper work.	Accountable to several Federal, state & local agencies; much paper work

Goals of the rehabilitation systems, or expected client outcome, is one area of contrast despite the fact that both the United States and Israel may share the same conceptual understanding of rehabilitation. Israel has legitimized what is in the United States a conflict of values regarding desired rehabilitation outcome. In the United States, work and more specifically work in the open labour market is *the* desired outcome of the rehabilitation process. In Israel, work is *a* desired outcome among other equally desired outcomes, such as the social welfare (i.e. social acceptance and social competence) of the client. This does not mean that social aspects are unimportant in the United States; however, they are often viewed primarily as significant *means* for achieving the vocational *end* of successful competitive employment.

The relative autonomy of the rehabilitation centre is another area of contrast. In Israel, a local centre is not directly accountable to each national referral or funding agency. As a result, the demands and controls exercised by the political components of the rehabilitation system are limited to its own agency. The director of the Israeli centre is, therefore, relatively autonomous - the managerial and professional *boss* of his centre. In contrast, the American centre is more limited in deciding who is eligible, the nature of services provided, and the length of service delivery. Limits and demands come from federal, state and local laws, regulations, and standards as well as from the numerous referral and funding agencies.

The organizational structure of the American centre differs from that of Israel. In Israel, the organizational structure is largely non-hierarchical. All staff report directly to the director of the centre, thus placing an enormous load upon him since in addition to relating to his funding agency he has the full budgeting, programme, and administrative authority and responsibility. In contrast to Israel's typically horizontal organizational structure, the United States' centre is more characteristically hierarchical. The director primarily deals with public relations, funding, and interfacing where appropriate with an umbrella organization or board. The director relies heavily on the service directors for the daily operation of the centre. Supervising the direct line staff (i.e. instructors, foremen, evaluators), the service directors and sometimes the assistant directors are middle management and provide no direct service to the clients. As can be seen from this brief description, there are several levels of professional staff who intervene, thus separating the centre's director, who is responsible for overall policy, from the clients. These two contrasting organizational structures raise important questions concerning potential advantages and disadvantages regarding staff/client interactions, decision-making and lines of communication, staff burn-out and turn-over, and programmatic orientation.

Staff in the American centre are more professionalized and specialized than staff in the Israel centre. Baccalaureate, master's, and occasionally doctorate degrees in rehabilitation counselling, psychology, and special education are required for most of the staff positions in the American centre. In contrast, a baccalaureate degree usually in social work is generally required of the professional staff in the Israeli centre. This is in contrast to the preference for psychology, rehabilitation, or even a business orientation in the United States.

Specialization of staff roles is also much more prevalent in the American centre than in the Israeli one. Staff roles and responsibilities are clearly specified by function in formal, written job descriptions in the American centre. In Israel, by contrast, responsibilities overlap and no written job descriptions exist. The direct or indirect impact of the degree of professionalization and specialization on client outcome or on achieving the goals of vocational rehabilitation remains unclear. Florian (1981) calls for more specialized training of rehabilitation workers in Israel, yet there has been some concern expressed in the United States (Bryen, et al., 1985; Willer & Intagliata, 1983) about the dangers of over-professionalization and specialization of professionals serving disabled populations. Unfortunately, to date there have been few empirical studies to help clarify this issue.

Decision-making concerning client's programmes and problems, as well as communication regarding the daily operations of the centre, are quite informal in the Israeli centre. This may be due, in part, to the organizational structure of the centre and the relative autonomy of the centre's functioning. By contrast, in the American centre, communication and decision-making are much more formal. Federal, state and local laws, rules, and regulations as well as the hierarchical organization structure of the American centre are perhaps largely responsible for this formality.

The formality of the American centre is likely to be a manifestation of the constant need for accountability. Because of the many federal laws protecting client rights and guaranteeing fair labour standards, and the state and local regulations and funding procedures, much time is invested by centre staff in providing written documentation of compliance and accountability to each of federal, state and local agencies. As mentioned previously, as much as 50 per cent of staff time is spent in writing and filling in reports needed for documenting how staff use their time, what services are provided to each client, client progress towards the goals and objectives outlined in the IWPP, client production rates, and so on. By contrast, in the Israeli centre there is considerably less paper work due to less concern for written measures of accountability (in fact no Hebrew words exists for the American concept of accountability) and more of an assumption that service delivery is a *benevolent effort which relies on staff's and management's good faith and dedication* (Bryen, Yaron, & Gozali, 1979). This factor contributes to the differing management and interactional styles extant in each centre - more formal and formalized in the American centre in contrast to a less formal and more personal style in the Israeli centre.

Noticeable differences between the American and the Israeli vocational rehabilitation centres have been described in relationship to desired client outcome, organizational structure and staffing patterns, and management styles. While these differences are noticeable, the question is whether these differences are also noteworthy. What effects, if any, do these differences have on clients?

IMPLICATIONS FOR CLIENTS

Here we enter the realm of educated speculation because, as we have stated earlier, few studies are directed at the relationship between system, structure, and client outcomes. Currently, a bi-national study which explores this relationship is being conducted by the authors of this chapter.

Some societal values and macro-system considerations appear to systematically diverge between the United States and Israel. Competitive employment is valued for its citizens in both nations. Yet social welfare goals have historically and cyclically vied with the traditional *work ethic* orientation for societal dominance in the United States. Israel, as a country preoccupied with nation-building, has an embedded religiously and culturally based work tradition of mutual help and humanitarian assistance. Thus it is likely that legitimate client outcomes in Israel will reflect this work tradition, viewing competitive employment as only one, among other, equally valued outcomes. In the United States, however, as society shifts towards or away from the primacy of either social welfare goals or the *work ethic*, so will desired client outcome shift in that direction.

The United States has a strong tradition of family primacy which is reflected in civil aspects of its legal system, but has very little legislated public policy which explicitly affirms the family's supremacy. Simultaneously, the United States has a strong individualistic legacy which is reflected in social legislation including its rehabilitation policies and programmes. In Israel, loyalty to the group and family are strongly embedded attributes which find their way into social, educational, and welfare policies and programmes. As such client outcome in Israel will reflect not only what is important to the client, but what is in the best interest of the family as an integral group. In contrast, in America, client outcome will be more focused on what is perceived to be *in the best interest of the client*.

The vocational rehabilitation system in the United States reflects these value preferences, and yet despite the overall lack of coherence among its many programmes still manages to regularize, individualize, and hold programmatically accountable the providers serving clients within the various frameworks. Facilities serving clients are bound by explicit rules of eligibility, service provision, individualized programme plans, and grievance procedures. The basis for these procedures is frequently found in federal and state legislation and regulation. In Israel, clients receiving vocational rehabilitation services are tied more closely to the predilections of the counsellors, trainers and administrators who deal with them at the agency or centre level. As such Israeli clients have less recourse through legislatively and judicially imposed mandates or other written procedures based upon explicit public policy.

Population, unemployment rates, and the mix of business-industrial enterprises surrounding a vocational rehabilitation centre do not appear to affect client outcome at the respective centres studied in this chapter. The centres' stated goals appear to be more significant for

179

impact on client outcome. In Israel the dual goals of return to the work force and the enhancement of personal adjustment and acceptance are contrasted with the primary goal of the American centre of successful employment in the open labour market. Although analysts might make a case for the dangers of overemphasizing semantic distinctions, real differences do exist. The main goal of the American vocational rehabilitation centre is to place eligible clients in competitive employment. An acceptable, if not *the* major goal of the Israeli centre is the client's social integration in community, family, and with one's peers. This distinction may not be observed in all centres with similar structural and client characteristics in the United States and Israel. However, if a trend were to be discerned, vocationally oriented centres in the United States would more closely adhere to the primacy of the competitive employment outcome - if only as a reflection of their referring agencies' policies.

The nonhierarchical organizational structure of the Israeli centre produces a close-knit and more personalized client service and may help the client to feel more involved in the rehabilitation process. However, because of this structure, one could argue that a client may also be treated more arbitrarily and with less recourse to explicitly shared rules under which he/she might have recourse if rights or wishes were overlooked.

Finally, the staff in the Israeli centre are not as specialized or professionalized as their American counterparts. Specialization and professionalized interdisciplinary techniques are viewed as a major American contribution to the provision of vocational rehabilitation services. Individualized written rehabilitation plans ideally draw on professional resources and techniques available within the centre and the surrounding community. When applied in a timely and well integrated manner the potential for achieving individual client goals is enhanced. In Israel, staff, consisting mainly of baccalaureate level social workers provide largely unspecialized assistance in each functional component of the centre's operation. Israeli vocational rehabilitation leaders have been seeking assistance from Western nations, especially the United States, to increase their professional skills, techniques, and specialized trained manpower to more closely resemble these overseas' programmes. Importing specialized approaches may improve some aspects of the services delivered to Israeli clients. They will not humanize or necessarily make staff more responsive to viewing a client as a *whole person* with a complex set of personal needs and aspirations.

In summary, client outcome is influenced by macro-system considerations (i.e. the political environment of the rehabilitation system), and by the goals, organizational structure, staffing patterns, and management styles of the vocational rehabilitation centres. Unfortunately, the exact nature of this influence and its direct impact on clients is yet to be studied. In the final analysis, vocational rehabilitation is a human enterprise which impacts handicapped persons while simultaneously reflecting the societal values of which it is a part.

REFERENCES

Bolton, R. (ed.) (1976) *Handbook of Measurement and Evaluation: Rehabilitation*, University Park Press, Baltimore, Maryland.

Bryen, D. N., Yaron, A. & Gozali, J. (1979) *Services to the Handicapped: A Cross-Cultural Perspective of Services in Israel*, Technical Report, Temple University, Philadelphia, Pennsylvania.

Bryen, D. N., Reiter, S. & Newman, E. (1985) 'Services to the Mentally Retarded: A Cross-National Perspective,' *Special Education and Rehabilitation*, *1*(1), July, 1-39.

Florian, V. (1981) 'The Evaluation of Successful Rehabilitation Outcomes by Rehabilitation Workers of Different Backgrounds,' *The Journal of Applied Counseling*, *12*(4), 195-200.

Imershein, A. W., Chackerian, R., Martin, P., & Frumkin, M. (1983) 'Measuring Organizational Change in Human Services,' *New England Journal of Human Services*, *Fall*, 21-28.

Katz, S. & Florian, V. (1975) 'A Survey for the Organization of Rehabilitation Agencies in Israel,' *National Insurance*, 9-10 (in Hebrew).

Lorenz, R. J. (1983) 'Rededication of Placement? Fact or Fiction: Management Holds the Answer,' *Journal of Rehabilitation Administration*, *February*.

Willer, R. & Intagliata, J. (1983) 'Research and the Policy of Deinstitutionalization: Implementation, Evaluation, and Termination,' in N. R. Ellis (ed.), *International Review of Research in Mental Retardation*, Vol. 12, Academic Press, New York.

Chapter Nine

ADMINISTRATION AND MANAGEMENT OF LEISURE SERVICES FOR
DISABLED PERSONS: ONE EXAMPLE

Veda Beck-Ford and Wanda Fox-Smith

INTRODUCTION

Leisure is generally thought of in terms of *time,
activities*, or a *state of mind*. Each individual perceives
and approaches leisure differently. It can be positive and
contribute to feelings of satisfaction, pleasure and
creativity but just as easily it can mean boredom,
frustration and loneliness.

With the increase in availability of leisure time and
attitudes regarding leisure becoming more positive, the
pursuit of leisure activities has become one of the most
important means through which individuals establish a
balanced lifestyle and ability to cope with the pressures
and stresses of life today. It is an effective means of
improving *quality of life* and has the potential to increase
available choices in life. Leisure activities afford
individuals the opportunity to:

- develop and express themselves.
- develop new and/or different skills and abilities.
- expand or develop social contacts and friendships.
- promote family ties and relationships.
- increase motivation, independence, assertiveness and
  feelings of self-worth.
- experience pleasure and satisfaction.
- create and feel a zeal for living.

The negative aspects that some may experience are
generally a result of not knowing how to use leisure time,
the leisure resources available within each community or
their own inner resources.

It is what is done with leisure that is important.
Although leisure cannot be prescribed, a complete system of
services has been developed around leisure and what people
do with it. As Godbey (1981) states:

182

> *Leisure is not neatly confined to any one part of our
> lives or to any one social situation. You may find
> leisure by yourself, at school, church, clubs, shopping
> centres, in automobiles, tents, caves, in front of a
> television, behind home plate, in the formations of
> drifting clouds and in many other circumstances.*

Consequently a great number of agencies and organizations
with varying purposes and mandates have become involved in
offering various leisure services; leisure education,
leisure activities, therapeutic recreation services and many
more. Disabled persons are one of the consumer groups for
which services have been developed and are the focus of this
chapter.
     It is the intent of the authors to demonstrate how
leisure services and service systems can be coordinated and
integrated to facilitate the availability of a comprehensive
network of leisure programmes and opportunities for *all*
disabled citizens. The authors have approached the subject
from a broad community perspective so as to include all
types of leisure/recreation programmes and services;
therapeutic, educational and recreational.

FACTORS AFFECTING SERVICE PROVISION

Traditionally most services for disabled persons have been
provided by advocate agencies, organizations or associations
representing a specific group of disabled persons. For
example many local associations for mentally handicapped
people, and more recently the Special Olympics, have been
the primary recreation service providers for mentally
handicapped persons. Similarly local Multiple Sclerosis
Societies and local chapters of the Canadian Paraplegic
Association have provided some leisure programmes for their
members.
     Changes have been initiated in recent years in response
to consumer demand, financial constraint, enlightened
attitudes and an increase in research, knowledge and
documentation in regard to leisure and its value. As a
result the scope of opportunities in leisure for disabled
persons has begun to expand and traditional boundaries are
being extended. Evidence of this has been seen in several
areas. For example, groups and organizations whose mandate
is to provide services, other than leisure, began to
recognize that they can play a most important role in the
delivery of leisure services. Municipal recreation
departments recognized that they have a responsibility to
disabled citizens and responded to the demand for service in
a variety of ways. Agencies and organizations who have been
providing services to disabled persons for some time have

started to pool resources and join forces to ensure a full complement of services are available while making the most effective use of available resources, both financial and human.

Integration of disabled persons into community programmes and the right of disabled persons to utilize public services and facilities is becoming accepted as desirable and expected. Service providers at all levels have recognized that no one group, agency, organization or government department has all the resources necessary to independently offer all the services required by disabled consumers (*Freedom of Choice*, 1982). Finally and most importantly, the disabled consumer has recognized his right to freedom of choice in the pursuit of leisure and is becoming more assertive in his demands for service.

Hutchinson and Lord (1979) have a more global perspective, and have concisely summarized some of the changing concepts of leisure services for disabled persons:

Past	*1979*
few opportunities in recreation and leisure	*services in the community as a right*
voluntary advocate associations providing services	*provision of generic services by government, communities, and leisure agencies*
segregated programming	*integrated programming with support as needed*
extravaganzas and special events	*individual and small group developmental upgrading activities and experiences*
traditional, narrow opportunities	*wide range of experiences which meet personal-social needs*
recreation as a therapy	*recreation and leisure as an integral part of living and development*
leisure agencies primarily facility and programme providers	*leisure agencies providing adequate enabling and support services*

Past	*1979*
services based upon inappropriate values and ideology	*services based upon principles of normalization (e.g. small numbers, age appropriateness, dignity of risk, integration)*
professional domination of leisure services	*increased consumer involvement and control of leisure services.*

Many of the concepts which were only ideas in 1979 have now become a part of practice in innovative communities. A wider range and choice of opportunities can be found in 1985.

CONSUMER POPULATION IDENTIFIED

From the broad community perspective the disabled population includes:

- all age groups - infants through seniors
- persons with any type of disabling and/or handicapping condition
  e.g. mentally handicapped, physically disabled, visually impaired, learning disabled, hearing impaired
- persons at all ability levels
  i.e. a total range from the multihandicapped person who is dependent on others for most of his needs to those who are living, working and recreating independently in the community.

SERVICES AND NEEDS OF THE CONSUMER

Given such a diverse group of people, the range of needs to be met is indeed extensive. Even in smaller communities, where the numbers of disabled residents may be few, the range of services might, of necessity, be quite diverse in order to accommodate the unique needs of each individual.

If the leisure services available to disabled persons in any community are to be comprehensive, as has been suggested, all modes of service, therapeutic, educational and recreational, must be included.

Each individual should have the opportunity to engage in activities which are age-, culture-, and skill-appropriate and are consistent with the present level of social, emotional, physical and cognitive ability of the individual... The ultimate goal is for the

185

> *individual to respond independently to his/her leisure*
> *needs and engage in community-based leisure experiences*
> (Stensrud, 1978).

Numerous models of service continua have been designed by experts in the field in an attempt to illustrate the various roles and functions of leisure service providers and to provide guidance in the practice or process of delivering leisure services. A brief overview of some of these will serve to illustrate the broad range of services required to meet the needs of all disabled persons. The Sequential Recreation Model (Stensrud, 1978) is based on a developmental process. The components of this model are; Specialized Services, Transitional Services, Fully Integrated Services and it is sometimes preceded by Therapeutic Recreation. In summary:

Therapeutic Recreation: which takes place in an institutional setting, is segregated and therapist directed and is remedial in purpose.

Specialized Services: are segregated in nature, take place in either a specialized or community facility, preferably community, motivation is external and the programme is individualized to meet specific needs.

Transitional Services: provide an intermediate step between specialized and integrated services, take place in the community, ratio of disabled to non-disabled is fifty:fifty, are initiated cooperatively by participant and advocate of service provider.

Fully Integrated Services: participation in community services and are provided supports such as interpreters, transportation and assistance as requested (Stensrud, 1978).

Arsenault and Wall offer similar models of recreational participation incorporating several more intermediate steps into the process (Arsenault & Wall, 1979).

Hutchinson and Lord (1979) proposed a developmental community based model of which the essential core components are: Upgrading, Education and Participation.

The focus of the model is on:

1) personal-social development,
2) improving quality and broadening the focus of community services to include a wide number of individuals, and

3)   a community development process which includes consumer and parent participation.

Each of the three components should be occurring within the community continuously and simultaneously. A summary of the three components follows:

> *The UPGRADE component of the model involves the upgrading of skills and self-confidence of persons with disabilities and the upgrading of community services and programs which make participation easier. Personal upgrading can help minimize the differences between disabled and non-disabled persons. Upgrading of community settings benefits all citizens and ensures that integration will have lasting impact.*
>
> *The EDUCATE component involves the education of all persons involved in the integration process. This includes advocates in associations, recreational staff and volunteers, politicians, the general public, and non-disabled participants. Education about leisure and integration for participants previously not involved is also part of this phase. Both upgrading and educating are ongoing processes which occur prior to and during actual participant involvement.*
>
> *The PARTICIPATE component involves actual participation of individuals in community services and leisure experiences. Support and advocacy are provided in in egrated settings where needed and experiences are carefully selected to build upon participants' strengths* (Hutchinson & Lord, 1979).

The range of services outlined in these models is relatively extensive. Within each component opportunities need to be available for participation in a wide range of activities: sports, games, music, outdoor pursuits, performing and visual arts, dance, crafts and many, many more.

It then follows that within each activity type opportunities should be available for various levels of participation: spectator, recreational participation and competition. Even within these, varying levels of involvement can be found.

In summary, service provision to the population identified earlier requires a very complex network of services and service providers to meet the very divergent needs of individuals.

MANAGEMENT AND COORDINATION OF LEISURE SERVICES AND RESOURCES

There are many publications available which cover theoretical information regarding various concepts, methods and approaches which have been used in the management and administration of leisure services. Some of these are written from the perspective of managing municipal leisure services and/or community based leisure services while others deal specifically with service systems or models in therapeutic or rehabilitation settings.

Some of these are Recreation, Park and Leisure Services: Foundations, Organization Administration (Godbey, 1978), Creative Administration in Recreation and Parks (Kraus & Curtis, 1973), Therapeutic Recreation Service (Avedon, 1974), Managing Municipal Leisure Services (Lutzin, 1973), and Strategies of Community Organization (Cox et al., 1979). Other publications provide practical approaches for training individuals to utilize community services (Beck-Ford & Brown, 1984) or involving the total community in the process of providing services to disabled persons as outlined in Participation (Lord, 1981), and Mission: Recreation Integration (Alberta Recreation and Parks, 1983).

The common theme of these works is the need for a *planned* or *systems* approach to the planning, development, management and delivery of leisure services, whatever they may be and whoever is providing them.

A SYSTEM OF SERVICE PROVISION

Calgary is an example of one community which is attempting to meet the challenge of providing a comprehensive network of services for disabled citizens. It has taken the combined efforts of all service providers, the disabled consumer and various government departments to create a system which is effective in meeting the wide range of needs identified.

Calgary is one of a few cities in Canada which has within its Parks/Recreation Department a section whose mandate is to facilitate the availability and provision of leisure opportunities for disabled citizens. The involvement of this section has proven to be one of the key factors contributing to the advancement of services in Calgary. The section came about as a result of consumer demand and needs identified by agencies and organizations who provide services to disabled persons. The consumer, specialized agencies and organizations and other community service providers have directed the activities and development of services which this section offers. Factors which from 1969 to 1981 influenced the initial direction and approach to service delivery were:

1. A number of agencies/organizations were offering specialized programmes to disabled clients to upgrade skills *BUT* did not have sufficient resources to meet client needs.
2. Several agencies serving disabled clients saw a need for leisure services *BUT* had no mandate or resources necessary to follow through.
3. Consumers and agencies on behalf of consumers identified the need for community leisure programmes and opportunities but had no liaison or link to these programmes.
4. Disabled consumers became more vocal and assertive.
5. Personnel in the Recreation Services for the Disabled section initiated more active involvement with consumers and other service providers.
6. An advisory committee to the Recreation Services for the Disabled section was established to seek input from consumers.
7. A committee representing most disability groups was drawn together by the Provincial Social Services Department, to develop an ideal social recreation plan for the provision of service to disabled persons in Calgary.
8. The economy prior to 1981 was on a definite upswing and more dollars were available.
9. The Parks/Recreation Department gained approval from City Council to increase their responsibility for recreation services for disabled citizens through working cooperatively with other service providers in the City.

The economic recession experienced since late 1981, has greatly reduced the budget of Recreation Services for the Disabled as with all sections in the Parks/Recreation Department. Despite these setbacks, the section has continued to flourish. In fact, leisure opportunities available in Calgary for disabled persons have expanded as a result of encouraging and facilitating cooperation amongst and between service providers, sharing of resources and information, effective management and creative use of resources available and maintaining an optimistic and positive attitude.

The Parks/Recreation Department, Policy and Systems Plan adopted in 1981 established the role of the Parks/-Recreation Department as facilitation and community development. It also clearly outlines the department's responsibility and commitment to disabled citizens. With this support from the department and the citizens of

Calgary, the Recreation Services for the Disabled section has been able to develop creative and innovative services in response to community demand.

The remainder of this chapter will focus on the role of this section and its responsibilities to disabled citizens and service providers. This approach has been chosen as Recreation Services for the Disabled is the one common link amongst all other service providers in the community.

COOPERATIVE SERVICE DELIVERY

As the primary role of Recreation Services for the Disabled is the facilitation of recreation programmes and services, a diversified network has been developed to accommodate the broad range of abilities and interests of disabled persons living within the community.

The section works with individuals, community groups, associations, agencies, organizations, schools and health care providers to create a climate and attitude which encourages disabled persons to utilize community leisure services. The achievement of this goal involves:

> Public education - to overcome attitudinal and physical barriers to participation,
>
> Leadership Development - to prepare service providers and volunteers to facilitate the involvement of disabled persons,
>
> Programme and Service Development - to ensure an appropriate system of physical and social skill development opportunities are available allowing disabled persons to choose the level of involvement *in recreation programmes* which they desire.

Acting in the capacity of a facilitator and initiator, Recreation Services for the Disabled works in cooperation with service providers within the community to ensure the availability of a full range of programmes, support services and information resources.

The section itself offers a variety of services which assist other agencies and organizations in the development of their recreation mandates allowing for the growth and development of unique recreation opportunities. Support and information services available are:

Information Dissemination/Referral Services

- information is disseminated to the public and service providers regarding grants, programmes, services and training opportunities.
- information is relayed through a variety of means; inservices, regular publication of programme/service newsletters, quarterly interagency information sharing meetings and ongoing telephone contact.

Liaison/Consultation Services

- assistance is provided to agencies, organizations and others who offer leisure services to further develop the number and range of recreation opportunities available to disabled persons.
- liaison and consultation services are offered on a request basis and are available to all individuals and/or groups interested in developing recreation opportunities for disabled persons, providing there is a need.

Leadership Training Workshops

- assistance is provided to groups in the development and implementation of training workshops and seminars.
- assistance is provided to agencies and organizations in assessing needs and preferences in regard to leadership training and offering of workshops which address these needs. Workshops and seminars focus on upgrading the skills and abilities of programme leaders, students, professionals working in the field of disabled services, general recreation professionals and volunteers.

Public Education and Awareness

- assistance is provided through the coordination of public information displays and booths in the community, in services to parent groups and the public, and awareness presentations to day camps, school staff, students and community groups.

Accessibility Information

- information to disabled consumers, service providers
  and the public regarding the accessibility of
  facilities and programmes within the community.
- assistance is provided to other Parks/Recreation
  operations and community groups wishing to upgrade or
  renovate their facilities by assessing current
  accessibility of facilities and offering
  recommendations for revision.

Resource Persons and Information

- Recreation Services for the Disabled is staffed by
  persons with specialized skills who are made available
  to agencies and organizations upon request to provide
  current resources and programming advice.
- the section also has the ability to contract individuals with unique specialty skills in order to provide
  resources to agencies and organizations for workshops,
  seminars and training events.
- resource books, articles, and training packages are
  made available through a resource centre, coordinated
  and maintained by the section on an ongoing basis.

Integration Support Services

- a system of referral and support has been developed for
  use by disabled consumers and community service
  providers.
- support services are available upon request and are
  accessed through referrals, individual requests and/or
  others acting on behalf of the disabled consumer.
- the section offers a variety of education and skill
  development programmes to the public, disabled persons
  of all ages and recreation professionals within the
  community.

Calgary is one example of a large urban development
with many diverse leisure service needs. However, each
community within the city has a distinct and unique
personality, similar to those found in smaller rural areas.
The unique character of each community determines the
overall direction of programme and service development.
Experience has shown, due to similar consumer needs in both
large and small communities, that the planned approach to
service delivery utilized in Calgary can also be implemented
in smaller communities. Each of the services outlined are

designed to be flexible, reflecting the ever-changing needs of consumers, resources and community involvement.

PROGRAMME FOCUS AND SERVICE PROVIDERS

In order to manage the large, complex network of services and programmes necessary to meet the needs of disabled Calgarians, Recreation Services for the Disabled has divided its operations into three general service/programme areas.

1. Specialized Programmes/Services
2. Integration Programmes/Services
3. Hospital Support Programmes/Services

Each area has available the same services. However, how these services are provided or accessed may vary considerably, dependent upon:

- the consumer group to be served, their needs, interests and the current level of service.
- the mandate, structure, policies and procedures of the service provider requesting assistance or service.
- the level of involvement or commitment of the consumer and the service provider.

Figure 1 illustrates the three service areas, the services available, the primary service providers or *cooperators* relating to each area and the consumer groups being served by each area.

SPECIALIZED PROGRAMMES/SERVICES

As Figure 1 illustrates, the Specialized Programme/Service section primarily works with and provides assistance to agencies and organizations who serve a specific population of disabled persons or those which promote a specific activity. For example, the Calgary Association for the Mentally Handicapped, the Calgary Association for Children and Adults with Learning Disabilities, the In-definite Arts Society and the Alberta Association for Disabled Skiers provide the basic skill development programmes.

FIGURE 1 SUMMARY OF FUNCTIONS AND ROLE OF RECREATION SERVICES FOR THE DISABLED

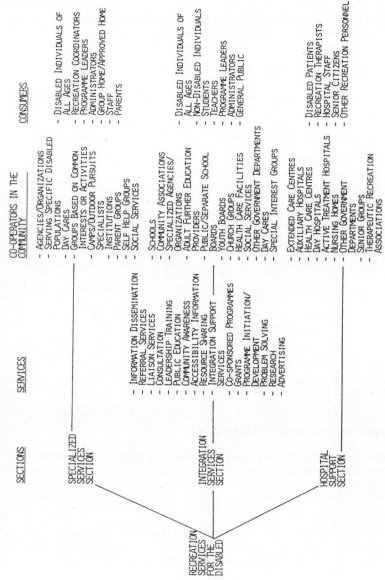

Examples of Programmes/Services

1. Co-sponsorship of Programmes

This service is intended to assist those groups who are providing specialized programmes, that is basic *learn to* or introductory recreation programmes specifically designed for disabled participants, to extend their resources and ability to provide service to their clientele. Programmes range from learn to ski, canoe, rock climb, swim, weave and paint, to programmes which enable participants to develop social skills, community and leisure awareness and a personal leisure lifestyle plan.

The assistance provided is based on the needs identified by the service providers as being necessary to extend and implement their programmes. Assistance from Recreation Services for the Disabled includes:

- provision of qualified programme leaders or instructors.
- payment of facility rental costs.
- loan of equipment.
- provision of programme supplies.
- advertisement of the programme.
- training of staff, leaders and/or volunteers.
- consultation with regard to development of mandate and/or programmes, applications for grants or other sources of funds, resources available and how to access them or problem solving and mediating.

The cost and responsibility of offering the programmes is shared by the service provider(s) involved and Recreation Services for the Disabled.

This collaboration results in the increased ability of service providers to offer programmes to their clients. Consequently, more and more leisure opportunities become available to disabled persons with less financial burden placed on the service providers and the consumer.

2. Co-sponsorship of Leadership Training Programmes

This service is also designed to extend the resources of service providers through increasing their ability to make available to their staff, volunteers and participants, opportunities to further develop skills and knowledge. As with Co-sponsored Programmes, the intent is that the cost and responsibility will be shared.

3.   Recreation Discovery Brochure

This brochure, compiled and published seasonally, provides a medium through which those providing *specialized* programmes to disabled persons can advertise and be assured of reaching potential participants. A broad and comprehensive distribution system has been established by enlisting the cooperation of schools, agencies, organizations and traditional advertising and delivery routes.

4.   The Creative Environment

The Creative Environment Project has been designed in an attempt to expand traditional recreation programme limits. Unique opportunities to explore and experience creative thinking, playing, and movement are offered.

The Creative Environment is, as the name suggests, a self-contained, lightweight, portable environment with ever-expanding possibilities for development and use. Within the walls of the environment, participants are invited to become involved in activities which encourage self-expression and imagination. Drawing, creative drama, dance, movement and story telling are but a few of the activities to be sampled and explored. A variety of story lines, costumes, scarves, musical accompaniments and other props have been developed as part of the project to assist in creating an atmosphere conducive to exploration, innovation, risk taking and fun.

Programme leaders are provided with a *how to* manual, so that the novice leader can utilize the Creative Environment as it is, or the more specialized leaders can further develop the programme ideas already in place.

INTEGRATION PROGRAMMES/SERVICES

This section was developed in response to the need, identified by disabled consumers, for expanded leisure opportunities in the community at large. To promote the active participation of disabled persons in programmes offered by generic recreation service providers, Recreation Services for the Disabled:

- attempts to ensure access is available to all programmes and facilities.
- offers a system of referral and support to disabled consumers.
- offers public education and leadership training.
- works with group home staff, parents or other persons significant to the consumer to ensure the consumer has

developed skills in preparation for involvement in a community programme.

Examples of Programmes/Services

1. Noon-Hour Recreation/Integration Programmes

Recreation Services for the Disabled collaborates with the public and separate school systems to offer this programme. It is designed to encourage the development of skills and attitudes necessary for play between disabled and non-disabled children and occurs over the noon-hour break within the school facilities. The programme is two-fold involving:

- Awareness Education - group discussion, disability information, activity preparation, and awareness activities.
- Integrated Play Programme - interest exploration, skill development, opportunity to develop friendships.

Cost and responsibility for the programme development, implementation and evaluation is shared. Programmes differ in each school, based on the student population, available resources and commitment of school staff.

2. Integration Support Services for Adults

A cooperative support system has been designed to provide opportunities for disabled adults in developing the skills necessary to independently register and participate in community recreation and leisure programmes.

Cooperation with the Calgary Board of Education, Continuing Education Department, Mount Royal Community College, agencies such as the Canadian Mental Health Association and others, result in the development of a network of services which offer support services to disabled adults, non-disabled programme participants and instructors.

Similar services are made available to disabled children and their parents, but utilizing a cooperative approach with various other children's service providers such as: boys' and girls' clubs; church youth groups; Parks/Recreation Department programmes.

3. The Awareness Team

Through the Awareness Team, Recreation Services for the Disabled provides a unique form of education and awareness to staff, participants, parents and volunteers, and the public regarding disabilities, attitudes and community recreation involvement. Each presentation is designed to match the needs, age and interests of the group requesting the presentation and includes:

- presentations and discussion led by resource speakers who are disabled.
- a variety of recreation activities which participants are involved in, while simulating disabilities.
- question and answer periods.

This service can be booked year round through Recreation Services for the Disabled.

4.   The Info-Mart

The Info-Mart is a 10-day travelling display initiated and coordinated by Recreation Services for the Disabled, designed to inform parents of disabled children and teenagers of the complete range of summer programme opportunities available.

Agencies and organizations providing specialized programmes, as well as those who offer integration opportunities, participate in the display. Opportunities range from a play programme for multi-handicapped children through to integrated programmes such as horseback riding and bike hiking. This is an educational approach in that it allows parents to see and understand the complete range of opportunities available for their children, in one place, at one time.

With this information, they can make an informed choice as to which programme would be most suitable to meet their child's needs and interests.

HOSPITAL SUPPORT PROGRAMMES/SERVICES

This service was designed to assist recreation departments within health care facilities with the development and implementation of their mandates, programmes and services, and to provide them with a link to community recreation services and programmes.

Support is made available by offering assistance to recreation therapists in:

- developing and carrying out needs and preference studies to determine needs of residents and long term development of recreation departments in health care facilities.
- offering co-sponsored leadership training opportunities for recreation therapy staff, programme leaders, instructors and volunteers and other health care staff.

- supplementing ongoing programme implementation through provision of resource personnel or experts who can provide information to upgrade programme content and teaching techniques and funding through demonstration projects.

Many more creative services and programmes are available through, or have been initiated by, Recreation Services for the Disabled. However, the preceding examples should indicate to the reader the range of involvement that a municipal recreation department can have in the overall system of recreation services in any given community. To facilitate this community development approach to service delivery, it is necessary to remain flexible and open to consumer request and demand. Emphasis is placed on cooperation and communication with any and all service providers. The system is designed to place responsibility for identification of need and provision of direct services on the consumer and the agency(s)/organization(s) working most closely with the consumer. The municipal recreation department in its facilitation role, using a community development approach, must be ready to be both re-active and pro-active in ensuring leisure opportunities are available.

WHY CALGARY'S SYSTEM IS UNIQUE

Calgary's holistic approach to recreation service provision for disabled persons is viewed as atypical. Certainly components of the service network can be found in other centres and many individual services are similar. It is the cooperation and communication which occurs amongst and between the many divergent recreation service providers which makes it unique. Each service provider, whether a health care facility, educational institution, agency, organization, club, municipal recreation department or one of the many others, has their own internal system or continuum of services designed to meet the needs of their participants or clients. It should be noted that many of these do not have recreation as a primary mandate, but recognize the contribution that involvement in this area can make to meeting client and community needs. Above and beyond the development of their own mandates, there is a concerted effort being made by most of these service providers to develop and direct their individual service systems to:

- complement, be preparatory to, or build upon services offered by other service providers.
- avoid duplication and, where common or complementary needs are identified, combine resources and efforts.

- connect or relate specialized services to integration services in an attempt to ensure a comprehensive continuum of services is available to all disabled citizens.

A very vocal, concerned and active disabled consumer population has been paramount in the development of the leisure services network in Calgary. Although needs and interests of various consumer groups vary considerably, there appears to be a common effort to attain recreational or grass roots leisure services. Opportunities to participate in and utilize community or generic services and programmes on an equal basis with other citizens is a primary concern, but does not preclude the need for specialized services. The type of support given and the demands made by the consumer have had considerable political effect in relation to development of recreation services.

Finally, the commitment that the City of Calgary, Parks/Recreation Department has made to disabled citizens, perhaps distinguishes its services from those available in other centres across Canada. The difference lies not so much in that a separate section has been created and established to advocate on behalf of disabled citizens, as in the role and mandate of the section, the size of the section and wide range of involvements and community links it promotes and maintains in order to ensure leisure opportunities are available to all disabled persons.

The fact that Recreation Services for the Disabled exists has been criticized by some, in the belief that a separate section perpetuates the segregation of disabled persons from the mainstream of leisure services. If the section were involved only in direct programme provision to only disabled persons, as exists in many other centres, including larger cities, this criticism could prove valid.

The *role*, however, of Recreation Services for the Disabled is one of facilitation utilizing a community development approach and does not provide direct programming to disabled consumers. A direct programming role would compete with other service providers and limit the scope of development and services available in the community.

The *size* of the section is significant. Many municipal departments even in larger cities do not have staff responsible for promoting or offering services to disabled consumers. Those who do often are limited to one staff person and a very small budget. This does not necessarily indicate that there are not a great many positive programmes and services being made available by these persons, but often their energies and resources are stretched very thin.

Currently, Recreation Services for the Disabled operates with a staff of five full time recreation professionals. Although each staff member has responsibility for a specific area of operation, a team approach is very much in evidence. All staff work out of a central office and their services are available on a city-wide basis, as opposed to a district or decentralized basis. Operating out of a central location eases access to services for consumers and other service providers. Coordination and communication is greatly enhanced.

The team work approach to service provision is the key to maintaining links between all the various recreation service systems in Calgary, that is, schools, health care facilities, agencies, organizations and many more.

All staff, to qualify to work in Recreation Services for the Disabled, must have a combination of both education - a degree or diploma in recreation - and experience - from two to five years' demonstrated ability in recreation and rehabilitation services.

As indicated previously, the *range* of involvements maintained by Recreation Services for the Disabled transcends or links all other recreation service systems from those providing therapeutic recreation services to those which support and enable disabled persons to take advantage of leisure services of their choice in the community.

Recreation Services for the Disabled has worked very hard to put in place mechanisms, such as consumer advisory committees and inter-agency information sharing meetings, that will encourage and support the cooperation found amongst most service providers and consumers.

POTENTIAL PROBLEM AREAS

Certainly there are difficulties and problems with maintaining such a service network. There are still some very evident gaps in service, both in leisure services and those relating to leisure participation such as transportation services and facility accessibility. The Parks/Recreation Department has committed itself to a steady program of facility upgrading to ensure barrier free access to all citizens, disabled and non-disabled to city owned recreation facilities. A majority of consumers have strongly voiced their opposition to the development of a large recreation facility, limited to serving only disabled persons and are in support of all facilities being barrier free with equal access to all. Economic realities, however, dictate that this is a long term process.

The system or total network of services is:

- dependent on a high level of communication and cooperation being maintained.
- dependent on each service provider maintaining their role or others being able to quickly adapt and respond to changes as they occur, in order to prevent service gaps or losses.
- dependent on one group maintaining the link amongst all service providers.

Further, there is no one controlling body throughout the system, therefore participation in the system is dependent on each service provider voluntarily *buying into* the concept.

DEGREE OF SATISFACTION WITH SERVICES

Preliminary results from a survey carried out by the Parks/-Recreation Department's Planning Section, indicate that other recreation service providers and consumers are supportive and relatively satisfied with the services being offered by Recreation Services for the Disabled and the community development approach to service.

The degree of satisfaction with services currently being offered was above 80 per cent. Data indicates there is less than a half point variance between the mean scores of what *should be* offered and what currently is being offered. Areas where it was felt Recreation Services for the Disabled should improve service or on which more emphasis should be placed, were in staging *special events*, supporting or carrying out leisure research and demonstration and in facilitating the availability of facilities for recreation activities for disabled consumers.

SUMMARY

It is felt that the system of services operating in Calgary could be implemented in any community, regardless of size. Certainly other cities have drawn from Calgary's system, ideas, programmes and projects and applied them in their own environments with a high degree of success. Similarly, Calgary has been able to implement and expand upon programmes and resources that others have demonstrated to be successful.

In summary, this chapter suggests:

- no one group, agency, organization or government department has all the services necessary to independently offer all the services required by disabled consumers.

- in order to manage the complex network of services required to meet the needs of disabled consumers and to co-ordinate the efforts of all leisure service providers a *planned* approach is recommended.
- in the community used as an example in this chapter, Calgary, success was shown to be due to:

  - cooperation and communication between and amongst service providers.
  - consumers having a strong voice in what services are delivered and how.
  - a strong support system provided by the municipal recreation department.
  - a concerted effort by all service providers to link their services wherever possible.

- the management and administration of leisure services in any community cannot be the sole responsibility of any one agency, organization, group or government department.
- the individual character of each community and the resources available determine what services are required and provided.
- it must be recognized that the roles and functions of each of the service providers and the consumer are equally important.
- flexibility, creativity and cooperation amongst and between all is the key to effectively developing a network of services and opportunities.
- an effective means of maintaining the system is having a common link to each and every service provider and consumer. Responsibility for this could be assumed by an interagency committee, a government department, or consumer groups.
- a consistent effort is required by this linking body to ensure services are initiated and maintained, gaps in services are dealt with, and consumer needs are responded to.
- an environment and attitude which encourages creativity, risk taking and a willingness to try new things will result in new and innovative practices in leisure service delivery.

Finally, the development of a comprehensive network of services is a long term, ongoing process. However, the Calgary example illustrates that this, in fact, is a realistic, attainable goal. The end result being that leisure services and service systems can be coordinated and integrated to facilitate the availability of a comprehensive network of leisure programmes and opportunities for *all* disabled citizens.

REFERENCES

Alberta Recreation and Parks Department (1983) *MISSION: Recreation Integration,* Recreation Development Division, Special Recreation Services Section.

Arsenault, D. & Wall, A. E. (1979) 'Service Continuum for Recreation,' *Recreation and Your Association: What Can You Do?,* Alberta Association for the Mentally Retarded, Edmonton, Alberta.

Avedon, E. M. (1974) *Therapeutic Recreation Service; An Applied Behavioral Science Approach,* Prentice-Hall, Inc., Englewood Cliffs, New Jersey.

Beck-Ford, V. & Brown, R. I. (1984) *Leisure Training and Rehabilitation: A Program Manual,* Charles C. Thomas, Springfield, Illinois.

Cox, F. M., Erlich, J. L., Rothman, J., & Tropman, J. E. (eds.) (1979) *Strategies of Community Organization,* F. E. Peacock Publishers, Inc., Itasca, Illinois.

Freedom of Choice, A Community Approach to Recreation Integration of Disabled Citizens (1982) A Campbell Post Produced film for the City of Calgary Parks/-Recreation Department.

Godbey, G. (1978) *Recreation, Park and Leisure Services: Foundations, Organization, Administration,* W. B. Saunders Co., Philadelphia/London/Toronto.

Godbey, G. (1981) *Leisure in Your Life, An Exploration,* Saunders College Publishing, Philadelphia.

Hutchinson, P. & Lord, J. (1979) *Recreation Integration,* Leisurability Publications, Inc., Ottawa.

Kraus, R. G. & Curtis, J. E. (1973) *Creative Administration in Recreation and Parks,* The C. V. Mosby Co., St. Louis.

Lord, J. (1981) *Participation,* National Institute on Mental Retardation, Publishing and Printing Services, Maple, Ontario.

Lutzin, S. (ed.) (1973) *Managing Municipal Leisure Services,* International City Management Association, Washington, D.C.

Stensrud, C. (1978) 'Sequential Recreation Integration Streams,' *Leisurability,* Leisurability Publications Inc.

Chapter Ten

ENHANCING EMPLOYMENT OPPORTUNITIES BY INVOLVING BUSINESS AND
INDUSTRY IN REHABILITATION PROGRAMMES

David Vandergoot and Edwin W. Martin

INTRODUCTION

This chapter presents rehabilitation administrators with an
approach to managing their programmes that will lead to
greater community support and increased resources to use on
behalf of clients. It is based on the experience and
research of Human Resources Centre (HRC), which is a large
education and rehabilitation facility in Long Island, New
York. HRC operates several, but coordinated programmes.
The school provides education to severely, multiply
handicapped students from infancy to age 21. Regular and
vocational curriculum are provided. Approximately 230
students attend school regularly. Efforts are made to
mainstream them into public schools when they are able. The
rehabilitation programme annually serves over 500 youth and
adults with all varieties of disabilities. Work evaluation,
training and job placement are the primary services.
Approximately 300 people per year are employed through
assistance from HRC. The research and training staff
conduct studies and develop professional training
opportunities for educators and counsellors that further the
capabilities of rehabilitation programmes. Abilities, Inc.
is a work demonstration project which shows how workers with
disabilities can be a part of a successful business
enterprise. Approximately 75 people with disabilities are
part of Abilities management and production staff. HRC's
basic mission is to improve employment opportunities and to
increase and improve educational programming for youth and
adults with disabilities. Working with employers to accomplish this mission has always been a cornerstone of HRC's
programmes. The knowledge and resources of employers have
been obtained for a very reasonable investment. This
chapter will describe the management processes that can be
used to develop working partnerships between the

rehabilitation and employer communities and the outcomes that can occur as a result.

It is important to focus on management because programme administrators are responsible for fulfilling a complex role with many functions. This is true of managers of programmes in both the private and public sectors. Public sector managers are often encouraged to operate service programmes with the same efficiency as private, for-profit goods or service producing firms. However, Drucker (1974) challenges the assumption that public and private sector managing is similar. He suggests that human services programmes bear certain burdens that businesses do not. The bottom-line orientation of most businesses defines a clear outcome to strive for. Human service programmes, instead, have to be responsive to a variety of value systems due to the support of competing special interest groups. Desirable outcomes, therefore, are less clear. Compromise may be required to support those outcomes which are acceptable to the most important programme constituencies. This may result in planning for less than optimal outcome for the group of individuals most in need of a programme's services.

These differing value systems might also influence how service processes are delivered. Such pressure often offends the professionals responsible for service delivery. Managerial stress becomes much greater when these circumstances exist. Efficiency may not be the means to survival for such programmes. Rather, a responsive and flexible management and staff is required to accommodate all the varied inputs that may actually be irrational from an efficiency perspective. A sensitive management system, rather than an efficient one in economical terms, seems mandatory. Managers must use this sensitivity to cultivate support among external groups.

Further support for this is the view that the forces which shape the supply and demand for not-for-profit services are different from those that affect the goods or services of the for-profit marketplace. Accountability is not nearly so difficult to achieve in the private sector. A business is viable if it can sell its products or service. Profits determine whether a company is efficiently meeting a market demand. Losses over too long a time a time can lead to bankruptcy. However, in human service programmes, the marketplace is subject to regulation by legislators, government bureaucrats, local pressure groups and others, often with little consistency.

These distinctions between public and private sectors appear to be eroding, however. Even the private sector is increasingly becoming socially conscious and politically responsive in spite of the costs that this might entail. The demands placed on managers of all firms are much greater than before and most likely will continue to increase. The point of this chapter is that business managers and directors of human service programmes, need to work with one another to be successful in meeting these pressing social demands. Vocational rehabilitation programmes are in a particularly good position to form cooperative partnerships with businesses because employers and rehabilitation professionals share the common goal of placing suitable workers in available job openings. Thus, external forces are creating a new situation in which employers actually may need rehabilitation services support. This view is quite different from the traditional one in which services to the handicapped are supported by charity.

The basis for this chapter rests on these assumptions:

1. Employers can use rehabilitation services for meeting their work force requirements and for gaining positive community recognition.
2. Rehabilitation programmes can use business leaders for gaining important community support for use with legislative bodies when public funding becomes threatened.
3. Employers can contribute a host of valuable resources, including funds, to help rehabilitation programmes become less dependent on public support.
4. Rehabilitation programmes can use the public relations expertise of business professionals to keep the local community aware of the value brought to society for its investment in rehabilitation.
5. Business strategies, including marketing techniques, are important tools for rehabilitation programmes enabling them to stay responsive to the needs of consumers of services.
6. Business can keep rehabilitation programmes aware of and responsive to changes in technology that, in the past, often have far outstripped their ability to stay up-to-date. This is especially important for those programmes which provide vocational skill training services.

The remainder of the chapter will provide guidelines for developing rehabilitation/employer partnerships. A marketing framework will be used to describe the concepts and activities a programme can follow. Empirical evidence will be provided to support the claims made about the expected benefits. A networking model will be used to explain how to initiate and maintain the partnerships. Illustrations will be given to show how employer resources can be applied to support a variety of services. Finally, examples of networking processes and benefits experienced by Human Resources Centre will illustrate these procedures and provide further evidence for the value of investing in rehabilitation/employer partnerships.

A fundamental caution needs to be made. A manager and staff can be so engrossed in developing an employer network that the network and its benefits become the main purpose rather than the means to the ultimate goal of placing people with disabilities into suitable employment. If the network and the resources derived from it do not serve the needs of these persons, it becomes superfluous.

DEVELOPING A MARKETING CONSCIOUS ORGANIZATION

The private, for-profit sector has developed a sophisticated approach to enable an organization to define its mission in terms of the needs of consumers who buy its goods or services. Perhaps this marketing approach is one strategy that rehabilitation programmes can borrow profitably from business and industry. This is so because a marketing strategy, applied appropriately, is a process that keeps an organization in touch with those who need it. Rehabilitation programmes, as all human service programmes, have an acute need for maintaining good external linkages. This is a result of the variety of pressures mentioned in the introduction.

The process a rehabilitation programme can use to remain sensitive to all its varied constituent groups can be described as a marketing strategy. Rehabilitation programmes have long understood that people with disabilities are a major clientele. Only recently has it been recognized that others are also in some way or other consumers of rehabilitation services (Spaan, 1983). Since society supports many rehabilitation programmes with public funds, managers must be sensitive to legislators of all levels of government. In this era of accountability and concern over limited resources, managers must have clear evidence of how rehabilitation is a social investment and have channels to those legislators who appropriate funds and devise laws affecting rehabilitation.

Managers also must recognize the diversity of referral sources which direct clients into programmes. Each source has its own reasons for using rehabilitation services and a unique way of relating to other organizations. Rehabilitation programmes can no longer respond to referral sources as if they were all alike. It is important to maintain good working relationships with a variety of sources to avoid too great a dependence on any one.

Other *markets* of rehabilitation have been identified as well, but the market receiving the greatest attention has been employers. Vocational rehabilitation has long worked with employers because only from them could placements for clients be obtained. However, employers were seen as relevant only at the end of the rehabilitation process and it was hoped by most professionals that clients would get jobs on their own. Indeed, research indicates that most rehabilitation clients in the area of physical disabilities find their own jobs (Fraser, 1978). Strategies have been devised based on the premise that it is much better psychologically for clients to get jobs independent of professional help (Salamone, 1971). Others, concerned over the fact that rehabilitation counsellors avoid employers, have resorted to placement specialists to manage employer contact while counsellors relate only to clients (Usdane, 1974). An empirically-validated technique, referred to as the job hunt club (Azrin, Flores, & Kaplan, 1975), was designed to combine the energies of counsellors and clients during the job search process. However, this model is almost always implemented half-way, leaving out, of course, the active role of the professional.

These approaches have been challenged by the idea that employers are actually service recipients of rehabilitation programmes (Molinaro, 1977). As service recipients, employers are a rehabilitation market. Various ways of serving the employer market have been proposed including client employer councils in establishing accounts (Ninth Institute on Rehabilitation Issues, 1982; Perlman, 1983). These strategies assume that employers have service needs of their own which can be met by rehabilitation programmes. This idea should have important consequences within a rehabilitation programme because a legitimate marketing strategy to employers will offer them services whether or not clients can be placed in their establishments. Marketing services to employers should not be an up-to-date euphemism for a placement service. In a subsequent section it will be shown that placement and related services are what employers primarily need and want. But their needs could extend into other areas as well such as for job modification, handling troubled employees and awareness training. Rehabilitation programmes serious about marketing strategy will be as responsive to all of these needs just as they would be to one of their clients.

Since there are clients, employers, referral sources and other markets to serve, it is important for a rehabilitation programme to be sensitive to different needs. Key to this knowledge is information. A programme must establish formal and informal information channels to all these markets. Not only are printed materials necessary, but personal contact is needed to ensure that accurate information is given and received. In other words, the entire organization must be seen as a system with a marketing orientation. Such a system will implement at least three basic processes.

1)   needs assessment of each market will be an ongoing activity.
2)   services will be tailored to meet these needs and will be revised, as necessary.
3)   personal relationships will be maintained with key market representatives by staff from all levels of the organization.

The next section will present the marketing approach used at Human Resources Centre to develop improved relationships with the employment community.

IMPLEMENTING AN EMPLOYER MARKETING PROGRAMME AT HUMAN RESOURCES CENTRE

Recent activities of HRC will be used to illustrate how the three basic marketing processes can be implemented within a rehabilitation programme.

Needs Assessment

Needs assessment is accomplished by conducting marketing research which can be defined as a way of gathering information to reduce the risk that no one wants what a programme is offering. Or, put positively, it is a method to increase the probability that a programme will be designed to meet a real need. Vocational rehabilitation programmes have a mission to develop employment opportunities for people with disabilities. At HRC one strategy to accomplish this is to develop relationships with employers. Therefore, marketing research was conducted to give information that would be useful in predicting with whom these relationships should be developed and how this should be accomplished.

A variety of marketing studies were conducted to provide some of the pieces of the puzzle concerning how to develop linkages with employers. The process of developing employer relationships is a complex one which can only be studied in approximations. A variety of methods were selected so that the knowledge gained from each could be combined to give a more complete picture of the process.

A second purpose of this research programme was to identify *market segments* or those different types of employers who would be more likely to develop working relationships with rehabilitation professionals and who can meet the needs of programmes and clients. It is useful to identify likely candidates so that resources and staff time can be used most effectively. Also, further market segmentation can be done by identifying employers who are or will be hiring, who have positions which rehabilitation clients are capable of filling, and who have locations accessible to public transportation.

The first study conducted was a survey of local employers. The basic questions addressed by this survey were:

1. Which employers are in a hiring mode?
2. Will hiring projections be increasing over the next six-month period?
3. Which employers provide on the job training? (Vandergoot, Swirsky & Rice, 1982)

Although answers to these questions are important in their own right, of more value was the process used to develop the survey form and create the methodology for conducting the survey. Six steps were used to conduct the research. These were as follows:

1) identification of expanding labor markets,
2) recruitment of employers to serve as advisors,
3) identification of relevant occupations in demand,
4) designing of the questionnaire,
5) identification of the employers to be sampled, and
6) follow-up with specific employers.

Staff persons did a preliminary review of published labour market statistics that were national and regional in scope. Occupations projected to be in demand were included in the survey to see if the local area had similar trends.

A second set of occupations were drawn from the skill training programmes already provided by HRC. It was at this point that several business people, well known to rehabilitation staff, were asked to provide advice. This group identified several more occupations for inclusion. They suggested how to design the questionnaire to insure its clarity and brevity. They also helped plan to which segment of the local labour market the survey would be sent. It was agreed that the 60 or so businesses most in contact with rehabilitation staff would be the target population. Since these employers were likely to be cooperative, it would be useful to know how they could meet the employment needs of HRC clients. Several were asked to identify other employers who would be candidates for long-term relationships. These new employers were approached by their business colleagues and asked to complete the survey as well. This identified new employers and tested their willingness to work with rehabilitation by filling out the brief survey. Those who responded favourably were followed-up by rehabilitation staff and nine of these eventually became part of HRC's employer network. This method enabled the staff to eliminate much of the trial-and-error associated with new employer development.

Other results of the survey were also useful. Two skill training programmes in new technology areas were begun as a result of apparent local labour market demand. These were a computer programmer training programme and an electronic test technician programme. Each course requires approximately six months of study. Students study in classes that include approximately 15 to 20 members per course. Placement rates from these have consistently approached or exceeded 85 per cent of all students who have graduated since the programme began. The results were also used in vocational counselling and planning with clients. Services were more easily tailored to local labour market requirements.

Services: This needs assessment study identified a group of employers who were likely to use HRC services to recruit, hire, and train clients. The next study was designed to find other needs of employers that could be addressed by rehabilitation services and to assess how well these needs were being met (Young, Rosati, & Vandergoot, 1985). Over 500 employers from various sections of the United States were sent a questionnaire. These employers all had used rehabilitation services and had what could be defined as a long-term relationship with a rehabilitation programme. The questionnaire listed over 27 services rehabilitation programmes could offer employers. These were grouped into the following categories:

1) placement services including screening and referring job candidates,
2) assistance and information such as providing job analyses and job restructuring consultation,
3) training services such as affirmative action compliance and co-worker awareness training,
4) training in occupational and interpersonal skills to potential job candidates,
5) follow-up services to placed clients, and
6) contact methods preferred by employers.

Employers were asked to indicate how much they used each of these services, how they evaluated the services, and whatever recommendations they could offer about the services. Approximately 150 questionnaires were returned.

The results showed that the most needed services were those that could help them meet their work force requirements. Over 90 per cent listed these services as the most important rehabilitation could offer:

1) pre-screening of applicants,
2) referral of job ready candidates,
3) work adjustment support to placed clients,
4) personal/social counselling offered to place clients in need of such support, and
5) availability of rehabilitation professionals through phone consultation, primarily to clarify follow-up needs.

Although employers felt that the whole array of services was commendable, the overall emphasis was placed on recruiting, hiring and maintaining workers with disabilities in the work force.

Figures 1 and 2 illustrate how this survey can be used to develop a marketing plan to employers. Figure 1 presents employer reactions to the placement services received from rehabilitation. Eighty per cent of the respondents used these services during the year prior to the survey.

FIGURE 1   PLACEMENT SERVICES

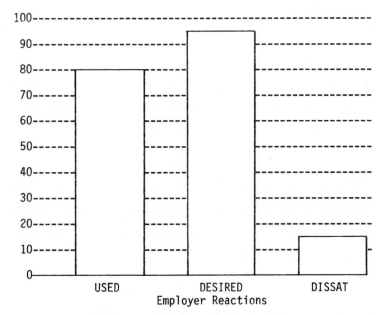

Employer Reactions

Adapted from Young, Rosati, & Vandergoot (1985)

However, almost a full 100 per cent felt they could have used these services. This suggests that much more placement activity could have been directed at employers with whom rehabilitation programmes already have good relationships. New employer development may not be needed until the hiring needs of these employers are managed. Also, almost 15 per cent of these employers voiced some dissatisfaction with placement services. In order to maintain good relations with this group, rehabilitation programmes need to identify what the concerns are and alleviate them. Thus, additional or improved placement services may be needed by about one third of the employers currently being served by rehabilitation. Again, this is welcome news as it is likely to be much easier to develop jobs with this group than with new, and, perhaps, unknown employers.

Figure 2 provides a picture of the reactions employers had to follow-up services which were defined as activities that helped a new worker maintain employment. Further instruction, counselling, transportation assistance among other services, can be offered during follow-up, depending on the specific needs of the new worker or employer.

FIGURE 2   FOLLOW-UP SERVICES

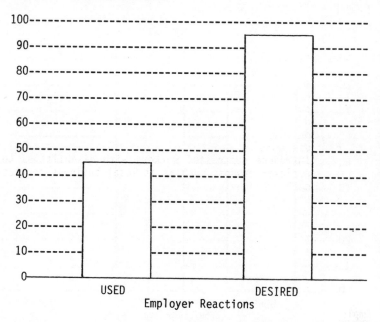

Adapted from Young, Rosati, & Vandergoot (1985)

Although the demand for these services is high (well over 90 per cent) only a little more than 40 per cent have actually been able to use these services. This means that more than twice as many employers who are currently associated with rehabilitation could be served in this way. Most rehabilitation programmes say they offer follow-up support but it appears that actual delivery is well behind demand. Failing to meet employer follow-up expectations may eventually erode good relations with them. Providing follow-up services more regularly may increase the job opportunities these employers are willing to provide rehabilitation clients.

Finally, these employers stated that all contact methods, including site visits, telephone, and written correspondence were useful to them. No one method was recommended over the others. They did indicate that phone contact was useful particularly during the follow-up stage after a client is hired.

After the survey was analyzed, a report was distributed to respondents. About 40 of them were able to meet in small groups to discuss reactions to the findings. Their recommendations to rehabilitation professionals for developing relationships with employers were as follows:

1) learn business jargon - talk the language of business;
2) visit local company sites that provide jobs suitable for clients;
3) gather background information on companies;
4) have employers visit local rehabilitation settings;
5) present rehabilitation as a marketing strategy for promoting the employment of people with disabilities - show how employing clients will meet the employer's needs;
6) use success stories to illustrate the potential. Introduce successful workers with disabilities to employer groups, such as at local business service club meetings;
7) be honest - when reviewing a client for an opening with an employer present all facts, positive and negative;
8) help co-workers and supervisors become comfortable with working with a person with a disability;
9) consolidate local rehabilitation efforts through a job clearing-house; and,
10) coordinate local rehabilitation efforts.

Employer Relationships: A third study was directed more at the process of building employer relationships than structuring the service programme most wanted by them. Fifteen programmes which had established advisory councils or networks with employers were studied in detail. These relationships were identified as partnerships (McCarthy, 1984). Programme administrators, staff professionals and participating employers were surveyed and interviewed during site-visits. The rehabilitation professionals pointed out that in most cases partnership networks can be created without hiring additional paid staff. Instead, re-assigning staff and using volunteers is sufficient to manage networking duties. Administrators concluded that building formal networking relationships with employers could be done with negligible costs. In return for this networking they listed these benefits:

1) additional community funding,
2) improved staff capability,
3) improved programmes, and
4) higher paying jobs and more opportunities for clients.

The rehabilitation professionals surveyed were consistent in describing how successful networks with employers were built. An essential first step was to identify goals that are shared mutually by employers and rehabilitation professionals. This always centered around the recruiting and hiring of capable workers with disabilities. Once a network started it was maintained by personal, informal and ongoing contacts between all members to build trust and friendship that created bonds ever stronger than the sharing of mutual goals. Network meetings, phone calls, lunches and recreational activities were all suitable contacts. Formal public relations mechanisms included brochures and directories, mass media announcements, network meetings and a network newsletter. Other ideas were to provide openhouses and awards to promote community recognition of responsive employers. Later in this chapter, more comprehensive networking guidelines will be described.

Employers gave two basic reasons for their relationships with rehabilitation programmes. The first included a variety of personnel needs such as the recruitment and hiring of good workers with disabilities. The second set of reasons was basically altruistic. Employers were sensitive to the needs of people with disabilities and felt a social responsibility. They did acknowledge that recognition in the community for this responsiveness was a valued incentive. Positive community visibility was a strong reward for many businesses.

McCarthy (1984) offered an important but overlooked point when he concluded that:

'while it is no secret ... that employers gain (in savings and qualified, screened personnel) from the vocational training and job-placement activities of rehabilitation practitioners, it would be wise for the

rehabilitation community to be more mindful and proud of this. The impression communicated by many rehabilitationists in the research was that they were gaining from the employment community more than they were giving. If this is true, they need to improve their resources and contributions; if it were not, that is hardly an advantageous posture from which to market services or negotiate a partnership'.

The approach that rehabilitation professionals use can be much more positive than it often is. Employers gain from their rehabilitation contacts and value them. The relationship is one of mutuality and not subservience. True partnership is possible.

The last study to be reported here was conducted to trace the development of rehabilitation/employer networks from their inception to a point at least two years later. This study permitted a determination of the successful establishment of a network, factors that related to success or failure, and the benefits that resulted from successful partnerships as compared to unsuccessful ones. Although not an experimental study, it is one of the few available that studied unsuccessful network attempts (Vandergoot & Swirsky, 1982). Available literature is derived almost exclusively from studies of only successful partnerships. A total of seven facilities in the State of Connecticut were studied as they implemented an employer partnership model. These partnerships were referred to as Business Advisory Councils (BAC). Five of the seven rehabilitation programmes were judged to have successfully developed a BAC after two years. The outcome was as follows:

1. Two of the successful facilities received increased community funding. Neither of the unsuccessful facilities did.
2. Four successful facilities received regular labour market information useful for counselling clients and making programme decisions. Such information was not available to unsuccessful facilities.
3. Three of the successful facilities obtained donated equipment from employers for enhancing skill training programmes. Neither of the unsuccessful facilities received this.
4. Three of the successful facilities obtained employer involvement in training clients' job search skills and developing placement plans. The unsuccessful facilities did not.
5. Four successful facilities developed community-based training slots in employer establishments. Both of the unsuccessful facilities accomplished this also.

6. All five of the successful facilities established new in-house training programmes which often were supported by curriculum suggestions and equipment by employers. The unsuccessful programmes did not do this.
7. Three of the successful facilities received management consultation from business people. One facility considered closing down until the BAC stepped in to guide a successful turn around. This support was not found in the unsuccessful facilities.

The cumulative impression from these studies is that the rehabilitation community and the business community have much to offer each other. Building employer relationships is possible and beneficial. Employers value the support of rehabilitation programmes for the recruitment and successful hiring of workers with a disability. Their needs for reducing employment-related costs and for community visibility are the bases for designing rehabilitation services for business people. A marketing strategy can be based on meeting parallel needs in both the employment and rehabilitation communities. The process of meeting each other's needs can be viewed as network building which results in close-working employer/rehabilitation partnerships. The key result of these partnerships is the improved employment opportunities for people with disabilities.

BUILDING SUCCESSFUL EMPLOYER/REHABILITATION NETWORKS

This chapter has referred to the process of building employer relationships as networking. Naisbitt (1982) provides a useful definition of networking as

> *'... people talking to each other, sharing ideas, information and resources. The point is often made that networking is a verb, not a noun. The important part is not the network, the finished product, but the process of getting there - the communication that creates linkages between people and clusters of people.'*

The key point is that networking is a process. If a network stops being a process, it ceases to exist. A network is a vehicle for communicating information. The current rate of rapid change requires that new information transmission structures be built. Networks are a structural response to information overload. Networks provide a series of channels for people to communicate with each other.

Human Resources Centre has applied what was learned from the marketing research and from additional experience gained from developing and maintaining Business Advisory

Councils to help other communities across the United States form and maintain employer/rehabilitation partnerships (Vandergoot, 1982). The approach taken was to help rehabilitation programmes form a network before formal attempts were made to include employers. There are several reasons for developing the rehabilitation community first. As the research pointed out and as many employers confirm, they prefer to work with a coordinated network rather than individually with each rehabilitation programme. This reduces time and effort. Also, the rehabilitation programmes in a community are all trying to do essentially the same thing. It makes sense to consolidate efforts and resources in the achievement of a common goal.

Besides managing and communicating information, networks provide other benefits. The rehabilitation community generally perceives that resources for providing services are scarce. If this is so, professionals need to be aware of the competition for these scarce resources. Networks can perceive threats to funding and organize a concerted effort to ensure continued and adequate support.

Another economic reason for networking is to distribute resources equitably across the community of rehabilitation programmes. A fair distribution can address the full array of needs of rehabilitation clients.

Networks also permit an opportunity for leaders of the rehabilitation community to work on eliminating the competition for funds, clients, and employers that so often exists among rehabilitation programmes. This competition leads to duplication of services and a tarnished image in the eyes of the community.

It has already been noted that rehabilitation administrators find the costs of networking to be minimal. One of the reasons for this is that networking can lead to bartering of resources including job leads, employer contacts, and staff.

Networks permit community-wide problem solving. Any one programme, acting alone, may be unable to solve difficult problems such as a lack of job opening for clients, keeping training equipment up-to-date with modern technology, or a transportation system that is ill-equipped to bring persons with a disability back and forth to work. Facing these problems alone can breed a defeatist attitude. Working as a network can create an awareness of the strengths that can be combined to overcome barriers such as these. The motivation resulting from working together is in itself not an unsubstantial resource. In this way, strengths can be recognized and shared.

In spite of all these reasons for networking and all the possible results as described earlier, rehabilitation professionals rarely network with each other. It has been shown that employers prefer to deal with a centralized clearinghouse for placing job orders, yet even such a limited network as this is difficult for rehabilitation programmes to form. The typical response of each programme is to try and *out-do* the others. Employers become confused by this competition amongst programmes which, purportedly, attempt to do the same thing - rehabilitate people with disabilities.

Even if rehabilitation administrators agree to form networks many other obstacles still must be overcome. If a network is opposed by a powerful community group it is not likely to continue. For example, some networks have not been able to progress because the state-supported agency for one reason or another would not participate. Without state agency involvement, rehabilitation networks are not likely to succeed. In a similar manner, a rehabilitation network without employers is not going to work either. Another problem is that some people only represent themselves in networks and not their organizations. They want to be in a network because they believe it is important. However, their institutions may not necessarily support them. Members have to be able to mobilizee their organizations on behalf of the network. Individual representation is not sufficient to make a network successful. Organizations have to be committed to a network by empowering an individual to actually represent that organizations.

If a community group cannot see how it will benefit from a network it is not likely to be a good networking partner. Another problem occurs when an organization decides to join a network, but then does not receive the anticipated benefits. That organization will likely drop out and will not pursue networking, perhaps for a long time afterwards. Once a failure occurs, it will be much more difficult to get the group involved again. A careful, planning approach is necessary for networking. Participants must see how they are going to benefit and how those benefits will be delivered before networking can proceed.

There are some other general assumptions to keep in mind about networks. Everyone must feel that there is something to gain but, besides that, everyone must remember that there is a cost involved in networking even though it may not be very expensive. The common building block within a network is that everyone can build on strengths. Every group must commit some of their strengths and resources.

What do rehabilitation networks look like? There needs to be a balanced representation of community groups. In the successful networks that the Human Resources Centre has worked with there is no one group that dominates decisions. There is no one-way flow of power. For example, the state agency or a large employer will not dominate the network. Successful networks are very performance oriented. They do not have long range goals. These networks identify a current problem, figure out a strategy to deal with it, implement the plan which solves the problem and then move on to something else. It is short term and action oriented. There is an expectation that everyone will play a role with shared responsibility. Not everyone may do the work. It is probably best that not everyone should get involved in doing something because there may be too many people getting in each other's way. Sharing responsibility means sharing information, passing on a good word, making an introduction, helping set plans. However, the action is usually accomplished by a few key people. This distribution of activity affects the structures of networks. The structure must be very flexible. There is no need for long-term committees. Most of the committees are ad-hoc dealing with a particular problem. Member turn-over on the committees is fairly frequent. Typically, there is no real structure, no formal organization evolving out of networks. When a network becomes too formal it starts to become a separate programme with vested interests and competes with other programmes. A network is often thought of as a group of individuals coming together to communicate and to accomplish a common purpose. It can be represented as a circle with the word network on it. However, that is a wrong impression of a network. Although consisting of a core of individuals a network really is this core plus all the organizations that are represented. The true picture of a network would be a circle with connections to many other circles, which in turn, are connected to others. Every one should feel as if their circle was at the core of the network. There is really no end to the kinds of communication linkages that are possible. Another point not easily captured with this illustration is that a network is just never really completed. A network never stops growing and developing new information linkages.

There needs to be a caution here, however. There are some networks that have 300 or 400 people in them already. Typically, all of these people are not necessarily active in the network, nor do they need to be. Perhaps only 15 or 20 active people may be really necessary. But those 300 or so who have been involved in the past are always out there ready to be called on again. Actually, the burnout of network members usually occurs in less than two years. Network responsibilities are added to the regular professional and job duties of a member. Particularly if a person has been actively involved in accomplishing a network project, overload can occur. Plans must be made constantly to move people in and out of the active part of a network. Once a person is in a network, even though it may no longer be in an active way, that person is still accessible. Contacts can always be resurrected. New organizational representatives will need to be appointed on occasion.

Networks, as they grow, make deliberate attempts to develop formal communication links such as a newsletter, an annual meeting, or some other kind of mechanism to keep in touch with those people who had been active in the past but can no longer afford intense involvement. This serves to renew their ties with the network. The network should always be growing, and, given Naisbett's definition, if it ceases to grow, it may no longer be a network. The typical process that rehabilitation communities have used to develop their networks contains seven steps. Table 1 briefly outlines this networking process. In efforts to develop a network, it is first necessary to get the rehabilitation community together. This is not always successful. If initial collaboration among rehabilitation programmes is not possible then the effort to develop networking with employers is likely to fail also. If rehabilitation networking efforts are not successful, then the employer community will see the competitiveness and the duplication of services. They become negative to the whole issue of networking and even, perhaps, rehabilitation. It is unfortunate but in about half of the communities interested in networks that HRC has worked with, it was not possible to proceed because of a lack of integration among the rehabilitation programmes.

TABLE 1   DEVELOPING EMPLOYER NETWORKS

1. Organize the local rehabilitation community.
2. Start with a few good employers.
3. Convene a group meeting.
4. Problem-solving strategy.
5. Set up an organizational structure.
6. Initiate a pilot project.
7. Expand to meet identified needs.

Another obstacle to community-wide networking is that many of the varied agencies that represent rehabilitation within the community will want to set up separate networks. This intensifies the competition for employers to join the networks. The confusion created among employers becomes worse. In one city there were seven networks trying to develop at once. Networking can have a bandwagon effect. Everybody wants to do it on their own or everybody wants to be the leader of the community network. There needs to be a community-wide collaboration with no one agency playing the power-broker role.

Assuming the rehabilitation community comes together, the second step is to identify a few good employers. The first targets should be those employers who have had previous success with rehabilitation since it will not be necessary to convince them that rehabilitation is a good thing. To start, a network requires only six to eight employers. Since their history with rehabilitation has been good, there is no problem with having the employers attend an initial group meeting which is the third step. At this time networking is explained as a sharing of mutual concerns and problems, a setting of mutual goals, and the development of strategies to work together to achieve these goals. The different representatives are asked to describe the rehabilitation problems confronting the community. Invariably the concerns are about vocational placement. Placement is by far the central issue around which networking develops. This leads to the fourth step which is the identification, after several more meetings, of some strategy that will address the placement problems. Strategies have taken many different forms. In some instances a conference has been provided for employers and rehabilitation people to talk together. A media campaign or the development of a training programme that needs a particular labour market need has also been done. The strategies depend on the local problem and how the local people develop the solution. One thing that seems to distinguish the successful network is that the rehabilitation agencies involved recognized that the employers actually assume some policy setting functions for the rehabilitation programmes. If a network establishes a goal and requires different things from different agencies, these agencies must contribute what is expected. If that kind of a commitment is achieved, the success of the network is assured. The networks that have been the most successful are those in which the separate members recognize that the network has some policy setting authority. This is a particularly difficult barrier to overcome, but if members are serious about networking, they will recognize ahead of time that decision-making will be shared.

In order to accomplish any task, the network usually outlines a very preliminary structure. Developing an action-oriented structure is the fifth step. Usually ad hoc committees develop. For example, a committee may form to plan public relations. As soon as its task is over, the committee disbands. Good networks are very active. Members do not wait for things to happen. If there is nothing for them to do, they become inactive for a while. There is nothing wrong with this. Some rehabilitation professionals have felt that once a person is involved, he/she must be kept involved. At Human Resources Centre, several hundred employers are part of a network. For a while, efforts were made to keep each one active. This was impossible. Eventually, employers will back out from active involvement if they see no real purpose upon which they can focus. If their expectations about involvement have been raised but not met, they may drop out of the network.

If employers and others in a community feel they are needed, they will respond. They should be recruited for a specific reason. The network should develop on the basis of need. The first project is an important one. If that project is successful and gains positive publicity in the community, most employers will feel rewarded for getting involved. There will also be a much more credible foundation on which to recruit new employers and other community agencies. Implementing a successful pilot project is the sixth step. The seventh, and ongoing step, is to allow the network to grow naturally from its success. In terms of network expansion, growth also must be on the basis of need.

HRC has followed some networks for about four or five years. It has been found that the networks that have gone on for this long have run into certain problems. After things have gone well for a while, a network will face the dilemma of whether it should become a separate programme. This network begins to consider whether to offer services through its own mechanism rather than through the kind of brokering and facilitating that had been done in the past. This seems to be part of the evolution of networks. They tend to formalize and see themselves as a separate entity. Some have actually become a separate programme. Others have decided to continue the brokerage function. The outcome of these decisions is unknown. It would appear that setting up a separate programme defeats the purpose of the network. Also, after time, a network starts to be concerned about funding issues, particularly if it chooses to provide some services on its own. If it is to offer direct services, it will need a staff, office space, and more of the trappings of a formal programme. This will cost more and may lead to competition with existing programmes. Of the eight networks HRC has worked closely with over the last two or three years, three have decided to become separate programmes.

BENEFITS TO REHABILITATION CENTRES FROM CLOSE WORKING RELATIONSHIPS WITH BUSINESS AND INDUSTRY

There are a number of additional ways in which a rehabilitation programme can benefit from close working relationships with business and industry, amongst them the design and development of new or more effective training programmes, and the contribution of various kinds of support to the rehabilitation programmes from the business and industrial community. An example of programme design and assistance may be found in the operation of a training programme for computer programmers at the Human Resources Centre. In establishing this programme, HRC recruited a business advisory committee including data processing managers from banks and other companies, personnel directors of companies which potentially could employ disabled persons. Committees such as these have operated task forces working with the programme staff in a variety of activities including:

- helping develop a curriculum for the computer
  programmers and revising it from time to time,
- helping select candidates for the programme, and
- assisting in the development of a testing battery
  which would be helpful in predicting potentially
  successful candidates.

Still another group has worked with interviewing the students as they progressed through the training programme. This activity had two roles, first, in assessing the progress of the students and so becoming a part of an evaluation programme, and second, in helping acquaint the students with the kinds of questions they might get during the interviewing process with potential employers. Later mock interview activities and other kinds of role playing were also conducted using employers as well as programme staff.

Over the course of this programme the curriculum has been changed to include new programmes and methodologies that were becoming current in industry and that our business and industry advisors felt would enhance the employment changes of the trainees. An internship programme was also initiated with a number of the companies represented on the advisory committee which offered internships to strengthen the practical experience of the trainees prior to their first job placement. In a number of instances the intern stayed on in permanent positions with the companies offering the internships.

This programme has been highly successful as a result of the cooperation between business and industry and rehabilitation. More than 85 per cent of the computer programmers have been placed successfully over the period of several years and over 90 per cent of those programmers placed have stayed with the same company, often being promoted into more responsible positions. The business advisory committee members have been very active in hiring the graduates from the programme and in introducing the programme to their colleagues in the data processing field. For example, one large bank in New York City held an open house for data processing personnel from other companies (including competing banks) and at that time graduates from the programme were introduced and interviewed, various employers reported their experiences and, in general, a positive climate was created for the programme's graduates.

Cooperation with business and industry has been helpful in similar situations with other programmes. For example when evaluating a clerical and secretarial training programme and designing improvements to that programme, business and industry advice was important in introducing word processing and other technological improvements and in deciding how important or significant such an introduction might be, what kinds of equipment might be useful, and so on.

A similar example of support from the business community came about through the Centre's involvement in developing a national Industry-Labour Council (ILC). This private, non-profit organization brings together representatives from about 100 major corporations and labour unions in the United States for the purpose of assisting people with disabilities to find employment. It is supported through the member's contributions and by the Human Resources Centre. The Centre and its staff offer technical assistance and training to member industries and labour unions. The ILC staff offers information services concerning solutions to problems faced by the companies with employees who have or acquire disabilities. They offer workshops and training sessions, disseminate publications and hold an annual conference in which the industry and labour participants exchange information about their successful programmes and are exposed to new approaches developed around the nation.

Utilizing contacts developed through the ILC, the Centre asked the Honeywell Corporation for advice on developing its computer capacity. The Centre's needs included computer-assisted instruction for school children and for adults in the vocational rehabilitation programmes as well as in adult education programmes. Capacity was also needed for research and business operations. This request for technical assistance was generously met by the Honeywell Corporation and a design for a computer system that would meet those various needs was developed. More remarkably, the Honeywell Corporation foundation generously made a contribution of the computer equipment that was necessary to satisfy the plan. While not every company can be so supportive, it is not unusual in the Centre's experience to have companies offer support through either material or financial contributions, or through technical assistance and advice.

As part of the design of the new computer system it became clear that a new specially designed facility would be needed to house the computer and provide training space. Special electrical and cooling characteristics made this a complicated and expensive task. Once again the Centre's contacts with business and industry proved invaluable. The Chase Manhattan Bank, which had played an important part in the computer training programme advisory committee, headed an effort to build a computer suite using their own resources and those of companies with whom they worked.

This was a considerable support to the Centre and saved valuable funds for services that would have been required otherwise for construction.

Another example of industrial cooperation and help both to the rehabilitation facility and to the larger population of persons with disabilities comes from the Ford Motor Company. For a number of years the Centre has specialized in training people with severe disabilities to be able to operate motor vehicles. In addition to becoming the largest facility in this area of the United States offering these services, the Centre has been called upon to help establish programmes in other states and the Commonwealth of Puerto Rico. As our experience has grown, we have worked cooperatively with manufacturers in the design of special modifications for their vehicles including both automobiles and vans. Cooperative relationships in this area have been developed with the Ford Motor Company which have led to that company making available to us automobiles for our Driver Education programme, and our performing several research projects in cooperation with Ford.

One last example of possibility of support for rehabilitation activities from collaboration with business and industry lies in the area of developing actual work assignments for persons with disabilities. The Human Resources Centre has as one of its affiliate divisions a company called Abilities Inc., which is a non-profit organization designed to demonstrate the abilities of workers with disabilities in a variety of light manufacturing and information processing tasks. To operate Abilities, business is sought from various companies which is completed by staff of Abilities on a subcontracting basis. All employees are paid the minimum wage or more, and the work meets all of the standards of prevailing industry.

Frequently, contacts made through our placement activities with industry and through our technical assistance procedures lead to the consideration of Abilities for subcontract work. Although in the final analysis Abilities has to win the overwhelming proportion of its work by being the lowest or most efficient bidder, it has been helpful to have the kinds of contracts which give us the opportunity to present our bids to the appropriate manufacturers.

Finally, the Human Resources Centre like many other organizations solicits funds through its Development department to supplement government and other private funding. We have learned that the corporations working with us in training, placement and Industry-Labour Council activities are likely to respond favourably to requests for Development assistance. Many of our special events and special campaigns receive considerable support from the business and industry community that works with us on a day-to-day basis to advance the employment of persons with disabilities.

These are several and, in some instances, dramatic examples of assistance to the rehabilitation programme from major corporations. They are unusual because of their size and scope, but it is not unusual on a weekly or monthly basis for the Centre to receive assistance from one or more business and industry friends in forwarding its purposes. A range of information, technical assistance, financial and other support has been made possible through the networking programme which was basically designed to enhance the placement of persons with disabilities.

SUMMARY

The development of close working relationships between rehabilitation facilities and business, industry and labour, can be demonstrated to increase successful placement of capable workers, to strengthen and improve curricula and related training activities of rehabilitation programmes and to generate financial and other resources for the entire rehabilitation community. In order to obtain these benefits, managers of rehabilitation programmes need to consider these principles:

1. Rehabilitation programmes must accommodate the needs and concerns of a variety of groups, including people with disabilities, employers, referral sources, other rehabilitation programmes, legislators and government agency administrators.
2. An organization with a marketing approach will be sensitive to the needs of these groups and design goals and services accordingly.
3. Employers can provide many resources to be used on behalf of rehabilitation clients and are willing to become partners of rehabilitation programmes that actively implement a marketing approach to identify employer needs.
4. Networking strategies can be used to recruit employer partners and maintain their active support.
5. Networks should include, as members, as many representatives of rehabilitation programmes from a community as possible to ensure cooperation and efficient use of resources.

REFERENCES

Azrin, N. H., Flores, T. & Kaplan, S. J. (1975) 'Job-Finding Club: A Group-Assisted Program for Obtaining Employment,' *Behavior Research and Therapy, 13*, 17-27.

Drucker, P. F. (1974) *Management*, Harper and Row, Publishers, New York.

Fraser, R. T. (1978) 'Rehabilitation Job Placement Research,' *Rehabilitation Literature, 39*(9), 258-264.

McCarthy, H. (1984) *Partnerships Between Business and Rehabilitation: A Summary of Research and a Directory of Model Programs*, Human Resources Center, Albertson, N.Y.

Molinaro, D. A. (1977) 'A Placement System Develops and Settles: The Michigan Model,' *Rehabilitation Counseling Bulletin, 21*(2).

Naisbitt, J. (1982) *Megatrends*. New York: Warner Books.

Ninth Institute on Rehabilitation Issues (1982) *Marketing: An Approach to Placement*, University of Wisconsin-Stout. Menomonie, Wisconsin.

Perlman, L. (1983) 'Strategies in the Marketing of Rehabilitation: A Summary of the Seventh Mary E. Switzer Seminar,' *Journal of Rehabilitation, 49*, 14-17.

Salamone, P. R. (1971) 'A Client-Centered Approach to Job Placement,' *Vocational Guidance Quarterly*, 266-270.

Spaan, J. (1983) *Marketing: A How-To Book for V.R.* Dunbar, West Virginia Research and Training Center, West Virginia.

Usdane, W. M. (1974) 'Placement Personnel - A Graduate Program Concept,' *Journal of Rehabilitation, 40*(2), 12-13.

Vandergoot, D. (1982) 'Industry-Labor Advisory Councils in Rehabilitation,' *Rehabilitation Counseling Bulletin, 26*(2), 133-138.

Vandergoot, D. & Swirsky, J. (1982) *A Study of the Connecticut Statewide Placement Model.* Unpublished monograph, Human Resources Center, Albertson, New York.

Vandergoot, D., Swirsky, J. & Rice, K. (1982) 'Using Occupational Information in Rehabilitation Counseling,' *Rehabilitation Counseling Bulletin, 26*(2), 94-100.

Young, J., Rosati, R. & Vandergoot, D. (1985) *Initiating a Marketing Strategy by Assessing Employer Needs for Rehabilitation Services.* Manuscript submitted for publication.

Chapter Eleven

SERVICE PRIORITIES FROM A RESEARCH PERSPECTIVE: A PRACTICAL APPROACH

Gerry Evans, Jan Porterfield and Roger Blunden

INTRODUCTION

The opportunities to design completely new human service systems are few and far between. Even where individuals feel that they have such opportunities, they are often confronted with factors such as traditional ways of working and professional boundaries which quickly inhibit their ability to develop completely new systems. Boles and Bible (1978) have stated that the challenge faced by most institutional service managers is one of environmental repair rather than environmental design, involving an evolutionary process rather than revolutionary change. For those committed to such a process a major problem is often that of identifying priorities for attention. Failure to identify such priorities can often lead to crisis oriented service design which may not always be in the interest of service consumers, and can also lead to a lack of success, often quickly followed by disillusionment on the part of the change agent.

As a research unit which has a brief to develop services and to offer practical solutions to practical problems we are frequently invited into service settings to assist in the establishment of priorities and procedures for change. Because of limited manpower and time our opportunities to undertake such exercises are few in comparison to the requests received. On receiving one such request, it was decided to develop a model for service change, based on a research approach, which others could employ to achieve change within their services. The aim was to develop a method of establishing priorities for service development that could be used by frontline managers generally. Frontline manager is used to describe the person in charge of, and based within, the setting, e.g. head of residential unit, manager of day centre.

Managers of services appear to make frequent decisions regarding developments in service provision in isolation from either those who receive the service or those directly providing the service. Boles and Bible (1978) argue that this must be an ineffective method of planning since managers cannot be fully aware of the influences on service delivery in their service. *At best he or she (like everyone else) can obtain limited experiential and empirical information about some of the products and processes associated with the social subsystems* of the environment for which he or she has responsibility. Consistent with this argument, the principle underlying the procedures designed was that managers need sources of reference for establishing priorities and implementing the change required.

Hart and Risley (1976) stress the need for the manager to be responsible to, and supported by, *external agencies* who are concerned about the quality of the service which clients receive.

> *Just as staff work best when supervision is frequent, specific and positive, the supervisor too needs feedback, review and support from someone who cares about the quality of clients' living and learning experience. In particular the supervisor needs publicly referenced standards of quality so that supervisor and staff can join together to meet the criteria of excellence which represent no one individual's personal bias or preference. Standards are set by parents, by administrators, or by represent- atives of public agencies who refer clients and pay for their care.*

The arguments put forward by Hart and Risley are supported by an extensive body of literature which stresses the need for *counter controls* on human services, i.e. external controls which act in the best interest of clients (e.g. Boles and Bible, 1978; Skinner 1972). It is argued that counter-controls are essential in services for very dependent people (e.g. residents of psychiatric hospitals, nursing homes or mental handicap hospitals) who can exert little control on those providing services to them. These arguments have led to growth in the advocacy movement. Involvement of handicapped people and their families or advocates, in making decisions for improving existing mental handicap services and planning future services, (Department of Health and Social Security and Welsh Office, 1971; National Development Group, 1976, 1978, 1980; Tyne and Weirtheimer, 1980, Welsh Office 1983). There is therefore, a great deal of research and policy literature which suggests that services might become more effective if managers involve service consumers in reviewing service quality and planning for change.

Studies of methods of staff organization have revealed the need for managers to involve staff in decision-making. Raynes, Pratt and Roses (1979) comment

> *We have repeatedly shown that decentralization of authority, that is the involvement in decision-making of both direct care workers and their immediate supervisor, the building heads, has positive consequences for the care of the residents.*

Numerous other studies in the field of mental handicap (e.g. King, Raynes and Tizard, 1971), institutional psychiatric services (Towell, 1982) and business organizations (Hall, 1967; Paulson, 1974), have advocated increased decentralization of decision-making within organizations. These ideas have more recently resulted in the development of the *Quality Circle* method of participative management. Dewar (1980) writing about the *quality circle* idea states:

> *The key is participative management, and the approach should be encouraged from top to bottom of every organization. Responsibility for the quality of work should be returned to the worker; and he or she should be able to influence how the job can best be done. The worker's ideas and resourcefulness can often make the difference between success or failure of the best engineering concepts... Success is assured when participation is encouraged, because it results in a strong commitment to attainment.*

Therefore, it is argued that if a frontline manager wants to achieve successful change in an organization, his or her frontline staff must also be involved and must be able to influence, and come to *own* part of the change process.

These ideas form the basis of the method developed for frontline managers. It can, perhaps at its simplest, be seen as an extension of the *quality circle* concept by involving service consumers in planning services and collaborating with staff in service development. The remainder of this chapter will describe how such a collaborative approach to developing services was employed in a setting for mentally handicapped people, and will also present results of a monitoring exercise that was undertaken to evaluate the impact of the model.

THE SETTING AND PARTICIPANTS

Setting

The Mental Handicap Unit in which the study was conducted consisted of four bungalows and an industrial therapy unit. It provided long and short term residential and day care as part of the provision for the 325 mentally handicapped people of one health authority district, (total population 105,525). Two of the four bungalows and the industrial therapy unit were mainly used for training clients in preparation for transfer to community settings. A further bungalow was exclusively devoted to providing short term care for children with a mental handicap. The remaining bungalow, Bungalow 2, in which the study was conducted, provided long and short term residential and day care for adolescents and adults who were more severely retarded.

The researchers were approached by the manager of the Mental Handicap Unit who said he was interested in improving the way in which services were provided to the clients of this bungalow. In subsequent discussions the staff of the bungalow commented that they were unsure about what their roles should be, and how the service was to develop. Because the manager and staff were keen to make improvements, the researchers felt that there might be an opportunity to develop a method of making improvements which could be more widely used in services for handicapped people.

The Clients

During the study a total of 27 clients were observed attending Bungalow 2. Because many of the short term care clients used the bungalow infrequently, discussion of the results of the evaluative study will be confined to 14 clients who were observed frequently in the bungalow. Of the 14 clients, five were permanently resident in the bungalow, four attended the bungalow for short term care only and the remaining five attended for day care or a combination of short term and day care. Two of the residential clients attended school and the other three spent the day in the bungalow. The day clients arrived between 9:30 and 10:00 a.m. and left between 3:00 and 3:30 p.m.

The mean age of these 14 clients was 26 years, with a range from 15 to 64 years. Ten of the 14 clients were able to walk without assistance and 13 were able to eat independently. The group of clients had relatively good receptive language skills but limited expressive abilities. Six clients toileted themselves with only occasional or no accidents. None of the clients could dress themselves completely.

The Staff

Twelve Care Assistants worked regularly on the bungalow with two staff scheduled to work at any one time. Three of the staff had worked on the Mental Handicap Unit for less than a year and nine had worked at the Unit for up to three years (from the time the Unit was opened). Two had received a qualification for working with young children and all had received in-service training. Three senior staff were responsible for supervising the staff on this bungalow.

The Families

A total of 13 families participated in the study. These were the families of clients regularly attending the bungalow. One of the residential clients had no close relatives. Of the clients whose families participated, 4 received residential care, 4 received short term care only, and 5 received day care or a combination of day and short term care.

THE PROCEDURES FOR COLLABORATION

This section will describe the collaborative approach employed in the setting and will give examples of the changes made to the service as a result of employing the method. A more detailed description of the method has been written as a manual for frontline managers (Porterfield, Evans and Blunden, 1983).

The procedure introduced into the setting can best be seen as a series of steps which form a circular pattern of consulting clients, their families and staff; introducing new ways of working; examining the effects of the changes; discussing the progress made and making plans for the future. The steps are presented in the order in which they are followed.

1. Individual interviews with clients, their families and staff.
2. Planning changes in the service to achieve the required improvements.
3. Planning through joint meetings of families, clients and staff at regular intervals for the development of the service and review of progress.
4. Introducing the changes.

5.   Regularly monitoring the service to find out if the
      changes have been made and to examine their effects.
6.   Giving and receiving feedback on the ways of working.
7.   Deciding if the changes are effective in producing the
      required movements.

The researchers took direct responsibility for some of
the above steps while others were undertaken by the manager
of the setting with support from two other supervisory
staff. Having examined the time commitment required for
such an exercise, we believe that a frontline manager could
undertake the responsibility for implementing the procedure,
particularly if the opportunity for delegating tasks is
available.

Individual Interviews with Clients' Families and Staff

In this particular instance it did not prove possible to
interview the clients of the service because of their lack
of communication skills. While families can be considered
as service consumers, services should primarily be developed
for the benefit of clients. Therefore we feel that although
there may be difficulties in obtaining the views of clients
on the services they receive, it is important, wherever
possible, to develop ways of obtaining their views.
      Interviews were conducted with:

a)   all direct care, domestic and supervisory staff
      involved with the bungalow, and
b)   the families of clients who were resident in, or
      regularly attending the bungalow.

A structured interview schedule was used which enabled the
opinions of families to be obtained on their expectation of
the service and how successful it was in meeting the needs
of their relative and their family needs. In the case of
staff, questions were asked about the structure of their
day, any problems they encountered in their work, and also,
what they saw as being the aims of the service.
      At the end of the interview families and staff were
asked to select from the list below, three areas which they
felt were priorities for improvement in the services
provided by the bungalow. The list was drawn up by the
researchers following discussions with those involved with
the bungalow and informal observation of bungalow activity.

      Client domestic skills.
      Client contact with the community.
      Organization of staff.
      Client self-help skills.

Family-staff communication.
Client contact with the other bungalows.
Client recreational activities.
Other.

The areas for service improvement which were selected jointly by families and staff were:

1) Organization of Staff.
2) Family-Staff Communication.
3) Client Recreational Activities.

In addition to selecting the areas, interviewees were also asked to elaborate on ways in which they would like to see each area improved. On the basis of these comments, procedures were designed to achieve change in the three areas selected.

Designing Procedures to Achieve Change

Following the interviews, the researchers worked on procedures designed to achieve change in the areas specified by families and staff. These procedures for the three areas are briefly described below.

1. Organization of Staff. Staff organization was dealt with by implementing a simple method whereby between 9:00 a.m. and 7:00 p.m. members of staff were assigned to work with the group of clients in the lounge while other members of staff worked with individual clients. The nurse responsible for the bungalow assigned staff to work with either the group or individuals for one hour periods. A rota of assigned staff roles was prepared one week in advance and was displayed in a prominent position. If there were changes in staff during the week, the Care Assistants were asked to write the appropriate names on the rota.

2. Family-Staff Communication. In order to improve two-way communication between the staff and clients' families, a loose-leaf report book was provided for each client. The pages to be completed by staff were divided into three sections - morning, afternoon and night. Staff working during each period were asked to complete the appropriate section describing client activities. The individual client books replaced the existing method of daily record keeping for the clients. There were pages provided which also enabled the families to record activities when the client was

at home. The books travelled with clients between home and the bungalow.

3.   Client Recreational Activities. In order to increase client participation in recreational activities, each client was assigned a *key worker* (a member of staff with responsibility for particular clients). When the member of staff was scheduled to work with individuals, she was asked to spend part of this time working with her *key clients* on special individual activities. A leaflet describing the duties of staff assigned to work with the group, and a list of suggested special activities for those working with individuals was circulated.

As the above examples illustrate, emphasis was placed on developing relatively simple procedures which met the needs expressed in the interviews. The procedures were ones which were either directly taken from examples of good practice given in service literature or slight adaptations of examples of reported good practice.

Joint Meetings of Families and Staff

A family-staff meeting was held prior to introducing each procedure. A leaflet describing each procedure was distributed and discussion took place regarding the new procedure.

Before each meeting an agenda of items to be discussed was drawn up. It proved important that everyone present at the meeting understood that the main emphasis of the meeting was to discuss service issues rather than have a social occasion. Prior to the introduction of the joint meetings, the main form of contact between the staff and families had been at social occasions such as coffee mornings or fund raising events. At the first meeting it was stressed that the purpose of the meeting was to plan for changes in the service which would benefit the clients. Families and clients had to be encouraged to comment openly on changes which they wanted to see made in the service, and at the same time staff were made aware that comments made about the service were not personal criticisms of them. The role of the manager at such meetings was primarily to ensure that all involved understood each others' points of view thereby facilitating the process of change. The joint meetings can be seen as the focus of the collaborative system of improving the service.

STAFF ORGANIZATION LEAFLET

Special Staff Roles

An important part of your job is to spend time
with clients, making sure they have plenty to do
and talking to them.

Here is a way of organizing your work so that you
can spend more time with clients and know exactly
what to do at any time during the day.

One person supervises the group of clients.

Other people on duty work with one or two
clients doing activities and other tasks
such as cooking and bed making.

The Rota

There is a rota which tells you what job to do
for each hour that you are on duty. You will
be shown on the rota either as;

   G – supervising the Group
   or
   I – working on Individual activities

If you are working on the bungalow in addition
to the scheduled staff you should work on
Individual activities.

If you are substituting for someone on the
rota you should take over the roles indicated.

What to do

Supervising the Group (G): –

- put lots of different toys, magazines etc.
  in the lounge

- stay with the group (usually in the lounge)

- talk to clients

- encourage clients to take part in activities

- when a client finishes one thing give him/her
  something different

- praise clients for doing activities

(N.B. If only 2 CAs are on duty, the CA
responsible for the group may need to help with
things like lifting a client. If this is
necessary she should go back to the group as
soon as possible.)

Working on Individual activities (I): –

- do special activities with one or two clients
  (walks, cooking, arts & crafts, training etc.)

- do any necessary domestic tasks (making beds,
  preparing tea, serving meals etc.). Clients
  should help with these tasks.

- toilet or change clients who need help

- bring clients back to the group if necessary

- answer the phone

- talk to visitors

Introducing New Procedures

The new procedures were carefully explained to those who
would use them and others whose work could bring them in
contact with the bungalow or the clients using the bungalow.
Written information about the new procedures was given to
everyone concerned in the form of leaflets or pamphlets (see
example). These leaflets or pamphlets were used as a basis
for discussing the introduction of the new procedure and
were kept for future reference.

During the period prior to the introduction of the new
procedure, any new materials required were purchased, record
forms designed and printed and staff training conducted. It
was stressed that when the new procedure was introduced, the
front-line staff should be supported and assisted by the
manager and other supervisory staff. This involved
supervisory staff spending a good deal of time working with
other staff until they were comfortable with the new ways of
working. During this time slight modifications were made to
the procedures on the basis of the experience of staff in
their use.

Once the new change had been introduced and staff were
practiced in its use, supervisors reduced the amount of time
they spent with staff however, they continued to regularly
monitor staff implementation of the new procedure.

Regular Monitoring of the Service

A monitoring checklist was devised by the researchers for
use by supervisory staff. The checklist was designed to
monitor the extent to which the new procedures were being
implemented and also to identify some of the effects of
introducing the procedures.

During the period in which only the procedure designed
to improve staff organization was being implemented the
supervisory staff were asked to complete a checklist twice
daily. The checklist described the extent to which staff
were fulfilling their assigned roles. On the introduction
of the client report books questions concerning their
completion were added to the checklist. Following the
introduction of the third procedure the monitoring checklist
was expanded to include questions concerning client
participation in recreational activities.

FIGURE 1   STAFF FEEDBACK CHECKLIST

Date: ....
Time: ....

SERVICE AREA 1	1.	No. staff on the bungalow? If less than 2, why?	
	2.	Is the G supervising the group? If not, what is she doing?	
	3.	Is each 1 working with an individual? If not, what is she doing?	
SERVICE AREA 2	4.	Is there a client report book for each client present?	
	5.	Have all report books been completed for the previous shift?	
	6.	Are all reported activities appropriate and of value to the client?	
SERVICE AREA 3	7.	Does each client in the lounge have materials within reach?	
	8.	No. clients taking part in activities? No. clients in communal areas?	
		Record the names of each client in the lounge. Watch the G person for 10 minutes and tally each time she contacts a client.	Name 1. 2. 3. 4. 5. 6. 7. 8. 9. 10. 11. 12.	Contacts
	9.	Were all of the clients contacted at least once?	

Discuss this checklist with the staff.
Figure the client activity score using the Activity Calculator.
Put the information on the Feedback Chart.

This involved supervisors directly observing staff and clients, recording staff contact with clients and also recording the extent to which clients were participating in activities (see checklist). The supervisors were asked to complete each checklist twice each day which on average took 15 minutes.

Feedback to Staff

Each time supervisory staff completed a checklist they were asked to discuss immediately the results of their observations with the staff on duty. It was emphasized that they should do this in a positive manner, commenting on aspects of work that staff were doing well and, if appropriate, modelling or illustrating how some things could be done better.

A graph showing client activity levels and the extent to which staff were fulfilling their assigned roles was displayed in the bungalow. In addition the results were discussed at joint family and staff meetings and were reported at the weekly meeting of external professionals who worked at the Mental Handicap Unit (e.g. community nurses, social workers, consultant psychiatrist). To summarize, the method consisted of:

a) a process of consultation between staff and families of clients to determine changes that needed to be made in the service,
b) designing and implementing procedures to achieve the desired change, and
c) monitoring the effectiveness of the procedures and giving feedback to all concerned on the results of the monitoring exercise.

AN EVALUATION OF THE COLLABORATIVE APPROACH

While implementing the previously described procedures, the researchers also conducted an evaluation of the effectiveness of the method introduced to the setting. The evaluation examined the impact of the overall method on the clients of the service, the staff providing the service, and the reaction of families and staff to the developments. This section will be devoted to examining the results of this evaluation study. A detailed report of the results of the evaluation is available from the authors (Porterfield, Evans and Blunden, 1982).

Methodology

The study was conducted over a 24-week period with a further week of follow-up data being collected 14 weeks after the end of the study. Four measures were used to evaluate the effectiveness of the intervention. Two of these measures, the Staff Behaviour Measure and the Client Behaviour Measure were developed by the researchers for this and other studies. A manual, including details of the behaviour categories, observation procedures, data sheets, descriptions of the methods of summarizing the data and calculating inter-observer reliability is available from the researchers (Porterfield, Evans and Blunden, 1982).

1. Staff Behaviour Measure (SBM)

Using the SBM, the staff member's behaviour at the instant of observation was categorized on the data sheet.
The categories of staff behaviour were:

  a) Negative contact with clients (e.g. shouting at).
  b) Positive contact with clients (e.g. praising, hugging).
  c) Use of recreational, educational or personal materials (e.g. putting books away).
  d) Use of domestic materials (e.g. folding laundry).
  e) Administrative tasks (e.g. filling in forms).
  f) In office.
  g) Staff-staff interaction (e.g. discussing client plans, chatting).
  h) Other (e.g. supervising clients, drinking tea).

The categories were mutually exclusive. If the member of staff was involved in more than one activity, priority was given to the category nearest the top of the above list.
If the member of staff to be observed was not within the observation area at the time of recording, the category of *away or in private room* was recorded. If for any reason an observation was missed the *missed* category was coded.
While the measure allows for staff data to be summarized for individuals, the staff data for this study were summarized in group form only.

2. Client Behaviour Measure (CBM)

Using the CBM, the client's behaviour at the instant of observation was categorized on the data sheet.
The categories and sub-categories of client behaviour were:

I. Engaged

    a) Recreational or educational activity (e.g. painting, dancing)
    b) Looking/listening activity (e.g. watching T.V.).
    c) Personal activity (e.g. eating, combing hair).
    d) Domestic activity (e.g. washing up, dusting).
    e) Contact with another person (e.g. holding hands, smiling at while making eye contact).

II. Inappropriate

    a) Self-stimulation (e.g. rocking).
    b) Self-aggression (e.g. headbanging).
    c) Other aggression (e.g. pushing someone else).
    d) Other (e.g. swearing, stealing food).

III. Neutral

    a) Neutral only (e.g. standing, sitting).
    b) Manipulating materials unpurposefully (e.g. tapping pencil).
         Coding the neutral category excluded all other categories.

If a client was observed to be engaged and behaving inappropriately (e.g. doing a jigsaw while rocking), both categories were coded. If the client to be observed was not within the observation area at the time of recording, the category of *away or in private room* was coded. If for any reason an observation was missed, the *missed* category was coded.

SBM/CBM Observation Procedures

A detailed description of the observation procedures for the CBM and SBM can be found in the manual. For this study the following conventions were used. Observations of client and staff behaviour were made on five days of each week (Sunday to Saturday) for two hours (9:00 a.m. to 7:00 p.m.) for any one week of observations. Two 45 minute periods of CBM and two 15-minute periods of SBM observations were made in alternating order. (Either CBM, SBM, CBM, SBM or SBM, CBM, SBM, CBM). Individual clients and members of staff were observed sequentially at 30 second intervals. For reasons of privacy, observations of both staff and clients were made only in the communal living areas of the bungalow and not in the bedrooms, bathrooms or toilets.
    At the beginning of each page of client data, the number of staff in the observation area was recorded.

Similarly, at the beginning of each page of staff data, the number of clients in the observation area was recorded.

CBM/SBM Reliability

The majority of observations were shared between two researchers. Reliability observations were conducted approximately once a week (19 of the 24 weeks of the study) when the two researchers observed simultaneously but independently. The procedure for calculating reliability was the same for both the CBM and SBM. Reliability was calculated on the basis of each observation. Each interval may have contained a number of observation codes. For an agreement to be scored, there had to be agreement on every code within the interval.

The degree of reliability was calculated as:

$$\frac{\text{No of intervals on which the observers agreed}}{\text{Total no. of intervals}} \times 100$$

Reliability was calculated only for intervals in which the client or member of staff was observed, i.e. not for those coded *missed* or *out of room*.

The mean reliability score for the SBM was 93.9 per cent (range 85.7 to 100 per cent).

The mean reliability score for the CBM was 93.0 per cent (range 83.7 per cent to 97.6 per cent).

3. Research Checklists

Once the three priority service areas had been selected by staff and families, the researchers developed checklists designed to assess staff performance in these areas. The checklists were also designed to assess change in staff performance as a result of introducing new procedures. Information required by researchers for completing these checklists was obtained from bungalow records and by direct observation. Checklists were completed on each day that CBM and SBM data were collected.

Checklist Reliability

Reliability for the checklist was conducted on the same days as reliability for the client and staff behaviour measure when both researchers completed a checklist simultaneously but independently. Reliability was calculated on the basis of each checklist question.

The degree of reliability was calculated as:

$$\frac{\text{No. of questions on which the observers agreed}}{\text{No. of questions}} \times 100$$

The mean reliability score for the checklists was 94.6 per cent (range 81.8 per cent to 100 per cent).

4.   Interview Schedule

The researchers interviewed the clients' families and the staff before and after the intervention phases of the study using a structured interview format. Following the post-study interviews, each interviewee was asked to assess anonymously the usefulness of the procedures by means of an agreement rating scale. This was done to determine the impact of the intervention on family and staff opinion.

Sequence of Data Collection

The study was conducted in the following sequence:

- Baseline (4 weeks) - CBM and SBM observational data were collected.
- Interviews - interviews were conducted with staff and clients' families and priority service areas were determined.
- Phase 1 (4 weeks) - CBM and SBM observations were continued and checklists were used by the researchers to assess performance in the priority areas.
- Phase 2A (6 weeks) - the procedure to improve the organization of staff was introduced. Checklists and CBM and SBM observations were continued to evaluate the impact of the procedure.
- Phase 2B (5 weeks) - the procedure for improving communication between families and staff was introduced. Checklists and CBM and SBM observations continued to evaluate the impact of the two procedures.
- Phase 2C (5 weeks) - the procedure for increasing client recreational activities was introduced. Checklists and CBM and SBM observations were continued to evaluate the impact of the three procedures.
- Post study interviews - clients' families and staff were interviewed again to determine any changes in their stated opinions about the service and the impact of the research interventions.

As a follow-up, CBM and SBM data were collected for one week 14 weeks after the end of the study. To summarize, CBM and SBM observational data were collected over the entire 24 weeks of the study while research checklist data began to be collected in the post interview phase of the study. The agreement rating scale was completed by staff and families at the end of the study. For the follow-up phase of the study only CBM and SBM data were collected. Essentially, the study employed a time series experimental design with the individuals acting as their own controls (Baer, Wolf & Risley, 1968).

RESULTS OF RESEARCH STUDY

a. Research Checklist Data

The research checklist data was divided to correspond with the three areas targeted for change in the service. Data on staff compliance with the procedures was gathered by direct observation of staff at work, or examination of the client report books. The results are presented in terms of the proportion of times checked that staff were seen to be adhering to the procedures or had completed appropriate records.

Staff were observed to be following their assigned roles an average of 83 per cent of the times checked under the procedure designed to improve staff organization. In the case of the client report books, designed to improve communication between families and staff, it was found that on an average of 89.6 per cent of the times checked, staff completed the appropriate section of the report books.

Data on client recreational activities and contact with staff were collected from the period immediately after the interviews with families and staff. It is possible therefore to examine changes that occurred over the introduction of the new procedures. For example, in the post-interview phase of the study staff were on average contacting 55.9 per cent of clients in the 10 minute period observed, while in the last phase of the study, when all three procedures were implemented, they contacted 78.4 per cent of the clients in a 10-minute period. Prior to the introduction of the new procedures checklist data revealed that an average of 29.7 per cent of clients had at least one recreational material within reach while, in the last phase of the study, this had increased to an average of 73.5 per cent of clients observed.

The research checklist data revealed therefore that staff were generally observed to follow all the procedures designed to achieve change in the targeted areas for change in the service.

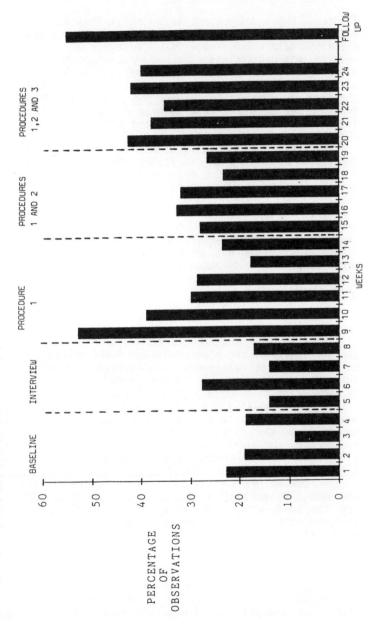

FIGURE 2 STAFF CONTACT WITH CLIENTS

b. Staff Behaviour Measure Data

Figure 2 shows the extent to which staff were contacting
clients throughout the study. The SBM data supported the
checklist data which showed that the degree of staff contact
with clients had increased following the introduction of the
procedures. The level of client contact rose from a mean of
17.7 per cent in baseline to 39.9 per cent in the final
phase of the study. Conversely the proportion of observations in which staff were talking to each other or were
involved in other non-client related activities fell from a
mean of 49.3 per cent to 27.2 per cent.
     Figure 2 does reveal, however, that the level of staff
contact with clients was variable. The initial impact of
introducing the procedure designed to improve staff organization, was that staff contact with clients increased
dramatically. This initial effect was not sustained,
however. An explanation for this might be that, while the
novelty of using the procedure combined with the support
received at the family-staff meeting resulted in the initial
increase, this was not enough to sustain adherence to the
procedure. This also suggests that the feedback procedures
used by the supervisors did not provide staff with consistent reinforcement. It was observed that the supervisors
were not consistent in their use of feedback procedures, and
therefore staff were not receiving regular feedback on their
work.
     When all three staff procedures were in operation in
the last phase of the study, a higher level of staff contact
with clients was maintained. The research checklist data
show that staff adherence to the procedures was generally
better during this phase. It is thought that the maintenance of the higher contact level and general adherence to
the procedures was, to a great extent, due to the increased
emphasis on the feedback procedures (i.e. more frequent
monitoring, immediate feedback to staff, public display of
client engagement levels, reporting of monitoring information to external professionals).
     Follow up measures of staff behaviour were taken, for
one week, 14 weeks after the completion of data collection
for the main study. As shown in Figure 2, staff were
observed to be positively contacting clients for 55 per cent
of the time.

c. Client Behaviour Measure Data

This section examines the changes in client behaviour
associated with the changes in staff procedures. Figure 3
shows the changes in client behaviour for all clients
observed throughout the study.

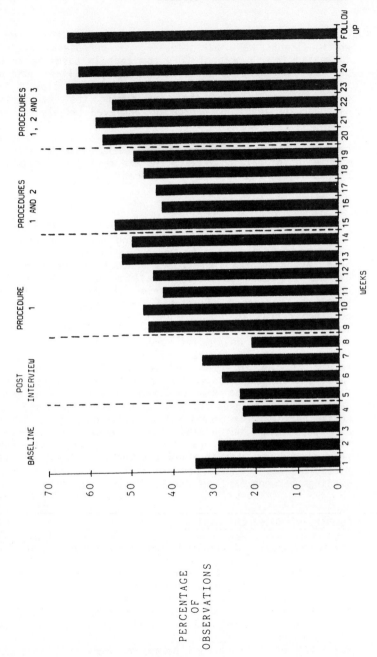

FIGURE 3 CLIENT ENGAGEMENT LEVELS

The level of client engagement (i.e. the extent to which clients were participating in purposeful activity) increased from a mean of 26.9 per cent in baseline to 59.5 per cent in the last phase of the study. Clients who were relatively inactive at the beginning also participated for a greater proportion of the time during the intervention, although the levels of engagement achieved largely reflected the skill levels of the individuals.

As shown in Figure 3 the follow-up measures of client behaviour which were taken for one week, 14 weeks after the completion of data collection for the main study, revealed a client engagement level of 65 per cent.

d. Rating Scale Data

Following the post-study interview, clients' families and staff anonymously completed a rating scale questionnaire. This was done in order to reduce any bias which may have been caused by the researchers conducting the interviews. Of the 14 staff interviewed, all returned the completed questionnaire by post, while nine of the eleven families similarly returned completed questionnaires. Results obtained reveal that the majority of respondents had seen improvements in the service as a result of the intervention.

There was unanimous agreement by all those who responded that Bungalow 2 staff were better organized as a result of the intervention. With the exception of one family, there was also agreement that communication between families and staff had improved. There was a greater variety of responses to the question concerning client participation in recreational activities. Three families were undecided about whether there had been an increase in client participation in these activities. All other respondents agreed that there was a higher level of client participation. There was overall agreement that the meetings between families and staff had been of value.

Summary of Research Results

The main results of the study can be summarized as follows:

1. Staff closely followed the procedures designed to achieve change in the targeted service areas.
2. Staff contact with clients increased.
3. The amount of time staff spent interacting with each other and doing other non-client related activities decreased.
4. The level of engaged behaviour for the client group increased with a corresponding decrease in neutral behaviour.

5. Levels of engaged behaviour for individual clients increased over the course of the study.
6. There was overall agreement by clients' families and staff that the procedures introduced had improved the services provided by the bungalow.
7. Changes in staff and client behaviour were maintained 14 weeks after the end of the study.

DISCUSSION

This chapter has outlined an approach that may be used by frontline managers to develop human services and has presented the results of an evaluative study of the implementation of such an approach. Because of the specific interest of the authors, the approach has been applied to a setting for people with a mental handicap, however, there appears to be no reason why such an approach should not be equally applicable to other human services. The key feature of the approach involved the provision of sources of reference to managers developing services, particularly reference to people with a direct interest in the quality of service received and those involved in the direct provision of services.

In the field of human services there was, and to some extent there still exists, the view that families have no desire to become involved in contributing to the development of services for their relatives. Certainly, it would be true to say that until relatively recently the opportunities for families to become involved have been very limited. The results of the work described illustrate a very positive response from families and this supports the findings of previous research (Cunningham & Jeffree, 1975; MacDonald, Uditsky, McDonald & Swan, 1976; Brown & Hughson, 1977). The families who participated in the exercise showed great commitment and often clear insights into the type of service they wished to see provided. For example, parents stated that services should not be content to provide basic physical care but should be continually stimulating and developing the interests of their handicapped relatives.

However, the balance of power in the relationship between families and service personnel is still often unequal and families can easily become intimidated and reluctant to comment on failure in service provision. It appears that only when there has been a shift in the balance of power will service recipients, or their representatives, be able to perform a role in monitoring services.

In addition to involving service consumers in planning, the procedure required the frontline manager to involve direct care staff in developing the service. In the setting where the approach was implemented a number of benefits were identified as a result of the involvement of frontline staff in the planning process. Staff reported that they had a clearer understanding of what their roles should be, and, of the goals that the service was seeking to achieve. The observational data revealed that staff had certainly changed their way of working following the introduction of the procedures. Comments made by staff also revealed that tensions which had previously existed between the manager of the service and the staff had also been reduced. This primarily appeared to have been the result of greater contact between the manager and staff and the achievement of consensus regarding the role of staff.

The regular contact between staff and families also proved beneficial in a number of ways. The negative attitudes that some staff held towards families were reduced as a result of greater contact and a greater understanding of the needs of families. In addition, staff quickly recognized the value of working collaboratively with families to provide a consistent approach in the client's home and service setting. In line with this approach, the work described in the chapter was extended by the service so that the needs of individual clients rather than groups could be examined.

The approach outlined for achieving collaboration in service development involves a series of steps that should be followed. The consultation aspect of the approach adopted in this study consisted of structured, individual interviews with staff and clients' families and regular joint meetings to discuss future service developments. The use of a structured interview method, in addition to enabling staff and families to select the service areas, provided specific information about the nature of the existing service and ways in which both staff and families wished to see it develop. The information obtained was invaluable in developing procedures which would meet the expectations of families and staff. The structured nature of the interviews also formed a good basis for discussing more general areas of concern to both staff and families. This type of comparable data, from a range of sources closely involved with the service, should be of value to all service managers.

The regular meetings held between staff and families were also important in developing informal contact between these two groups. Families in particular, stated that they found the meetings valuable because specific service developments were discussed. This required that each meeting had an agenda for discussing particular service issues.

A feature common to all the procedures implemented in the exercise was their simplicity. It is important to emphasize that the procedures were developed along the lines suggested by families and staff. The ideas for the procedures were obtained from currently available service and research literature. These ideas were adopted to meet the requirements expressed by staff and families. Since there are many reports of research findings and descriptions of good practice within services (e.g. Journal of Practical Approaches to Developmental Handicap, Mental Handicap, Journal of Organizational Behavior Management), it should be possible for families and staff to adapt such existing procedures for their own use.

An essential feature of the three procedures implemented was the regular daily feedback which staff were given by supervisory staff. The importance of such feedback was shown when it was noted by the researchers that regular consistent feedback was not being given to staff and consequently their level of adherence to the staff organization procedure fell. Feedback was important to both the direct care staff and to their supervisors. For direct care staff it was partly seen as an expression of supervisor interest in the work that they were doing, and when feedback was given in a positive way the experience of interaction between the differing levels of staff was rewarding in terms of staff relationships. For supervisory staff, the use of a structured monitoring checklist enabled them to enter the bungalow and focus directly on the ways in which individual staff were fulfilling their assigned roles. The use of this checklist by supervisors also provided a framework for discussion with staff about their performance.

In this study the researchers evaluated the success of the intervention in terms of changes in client and staff behaviour. The supervisors in order to give feedback to staff, also conducted regular observations of staff and client activity on the bungalow. The structured nature of the checklists and the regularity with which the supervisors made observations provided all staff with a simple evaluation of the effectiveness of the procedures implemented. On the basis of such data, they could make informed decisions about further developments in the service. This information was in a form which could be easily presented to families at the regular meeting. This would give families an objective way of monitoring the extent to which the service was being developed. Essentially it is argued that planning for service developments should be done on the same basis as planning good training programmes for clients (Houts & Scott, 1975) There is a need to involve all concerned in the beginning; to attempt realistic developments; to assign specific responsibilities to individuals and to regularly monitor progress.

SUMMARY

1. The approach described in this chapter provides frontline managers with a practical means of involving service consumers and staff in jointly developing human services.

2. The successful implementation of the approach for collaborative development of services has shown that the involvement of the families of clients in service planning is both feasible and desirable.

3. The results of the exercise have supported the findings of others who have argued for the full involvement of staff in making decisions about the services they provide.

4. There is a need for service managers to monitor and continually evaluate the services for which they are responsible. Such an evaluation should be made on the basis of direct observation of both staff performance and client behaviour and regular consultation with both staff and service consumers (i.e. clients and their representatives).

REFERENCES

Baer, D. M., Wolf, M. M. & Risley, T. R. (1968) 'Some Current Dimensions of Applied Behavior Analysis,' *Journal of Applied Behavior Analysis, 1,* 91-97.

Boles, S. M. & Bible, G. H. (1978) 'The Study Service Index: A Method for Managing Service Delivery in Residential Settings,' in M. S. Berkler, G. H. Bible, S. M. Boles, D. E. D. Deitz & A. C. Repp (eds.), *Current Trends for the Developmentally Disabled,* University Park Press, Baltimore.

Brown, R. I. & Hughson, E. A. (1977) 'Pre-Vocational Training for the Severely Retarded Adolescent.' *Journal of Practical Approaches to Developmental Handicap, 1,* 23-29.

Cunningham, C. C. & Jeffree, D. M. (1975) 'The Organization and Structure of Workshops for Parents of Mentally Handicapped Children,' *Bulletin of the British Psychological Society, 28,* 405-411.

Department of Health and Social Security and Welsh Office (1971) *Better Services for the Mentally Handicapped,* H.M.S.O., London.

Dewar, D. L. (1980) *The Quality Circle Guide to Participation Management,* Prentice-Hall, Englewood Cliffs, New Jersey.

Hall, R. H. (1967) 'Some Organizational Considerations in the Professional-Organizational Relationship,' *Administrative Science Quarterly, 12,* 461-478.

Hart, B. & Risley, T. R. (1976) 'Environmental Programming: Implications for the Severely Handicapped,' in H. J. Prehm & S. J. Dietz (eds.), *Early Intervention for the Severely Handicapped: Programming and Accountability*, Severely Handicapped Learner Program Monograph No. 2., University of Oregon.

Houts, P. S. & Scott, R. A. (1975) 'Goal Planning with Developmentally Disabled Persons,' Pennsylvania State University, College of Medicine, Department of Behavioral Science.

King, R. D., Raynes, N. V. & Tizard, J. (1971) *Patterns of Residential Care*, Routledge and Kegan Paul, London.

MacDonald, L., Uditsky, B. L., McDonald, S. & Swan, R. (1976) 'A Training Program for Developmentally Delayed Children with Behavior Problems,' Unpublished manuscript.

National Development Group for the Mentally Handicapped (1976) *Mental Handicap: Planning Together*, H.M.S.O., London.

National Development Group for the Mentally Handicapped (1978) *Helping Mentally Handicapped People in Hospital*, H.M.S.O., London.

National Development Group for the Mentally Handicapped (1980) *Improving the Quality of Services for Mentally Handicapped People*, D.H.S.S., London.

Paulson, S. R. (1974) 'Causal Analysis of Inter-Organizational Relations: An Axiomatic Theory Revisited,' *Administrative Science Quarterly, 19*, 319-337.

Porterfield, J., Evans, G. & Blunden, R. (1980) *The Client Behaviour Measure and Staff Behaviour Measure: Manual for Time Sampling Procedures*, Mental Handicap in Wales - Applied Research Unit, Cardiff.

Porterfield, J., Evans, G. & Blunden, R. (1982) *Improving Mental Handicap Services: Involving Clients' Families and Staff in Selecting Areas for Service Development*, Mental Handicap in Wales - Applied Research Unit, Cardiff.

Porterfield, J., Evans, G. & Blunden, R. (1983) *Working Together for Change. A Service Manager's Guide to Involving Staff and Families in Service Improvement*, Mental Handicap in Wales - Applied Research Unit, Cardiff.

Raynes, N. V., Pratt, M. W. & Roses, S. (1979) *Organizational Structure and the Care of the Mentally Retarded*, Croom Helm, London.

Skinner, B. F. (1972) 'Comparison and Ethics in the Care of the Retarded,' in B. F. Skinner (ed.), *Cumulative Record: A Selection of Papers*, Appleton-Century-Crofts, New York.

Towell, D. (1982) 'Developing Mental Handicap Services in an English County,' *Hospital and Health Services Review*, January and February.

Tyne, A. & Weirtheimer, A. (1980) *Even Better Services? A Critical Review of Mental Handicap Policies in the 1970's*, Campaign for Mentally Handicapped People, London.

Welsh Office (1983) *All-Wales Strategy for the Development of Services for Mentally Handicapped People*, Welsh Office, Cardiff.

Chapter Twelve

STRESS AND BURNOUT IN REHABILITATIVE SETTINGS

Sal Mendaglio and Doug Swanson

INTRODUCTION

This chapter consists of a discussion of job stress and burnout as they relate to rehabilitation agencies, individual staff members. This statement contains two important points which require elaboration.

First, while the manifestations of job stress and burnout are to be found primarily in the individual, their source and impact are to be found in both the individual and the institution. Second, both job stress and burnout are used intentionally to emphasize that these are two distinct, though interrelated concepts. At this point, it is sufficient to note that job stress and burnout are not simply synonyms.

BURNOUT: A HISTORICAL PERSPECTIVE

The history of burnout in the helping professions is normally thought of beginning with the publications by Herbert Freudenberger. Freudenberger (1974) first used the term to conceptualize the observations he made of the negative reactions of staff in an alternate treatment facility. Coincidentally, Maslach (1976) was concerning herself with negative reaction of helping professionals due to the interpersonal nature of their work.

And so, with the publications authored by these and others (e.g., Daley, 1979; Edelwich & Brodsky, 1980) a new area of inquiry was born. That is not to say that the phenomenon now accepted as burnout did not exist prior to the mid 1970s. The importance of these early publications rested in their drawing attention to this occupational hazard of helping professionals. As a result, the helping professional's *skeleton in the closet* was projected into public view. Such a conclusion is evidenced by the literal explosion of literature which appeared (and continues to do so) in virtually all of the professional journals. It is difficult not to encounter articles on burnout in nursing, education, and mental health journals. Further the popular media - both print and electronic - are equally saturated with documentaries and reports on helping professional burnout.

The phenomenon of burnout is not without its critics both in popular and scholarly periodicals. For example Time Magazine published an essay entitled *The Burning Out of Almost Everyone* (September, 1981). In one counselling journal authors both sympathetic to and cynical of burnout made their views known. One questioned the validity of the concept (Tiedman, 1979), another (Maher, 1983) noted that burnout was not only a new field of study but a new commercial venture - referring to the proliferation of workshops to combat burnout.

DEFINITION OF BURNOUT

Various definitions of burnout were proffered with the first wave of publications. It was common for a writer to begin with a reference to a dictionary definition of the term. For example burnout is *to wear out, to become exhausted*. With this initial approach to definition, analogies to burning were also common. More sophisticated definitions soon arose. Burnout was described as a syndrome consisting of both psychological and physical symptoms. A sample of these definitions are cited here.

> A burned out person is...*someone in a state of fatigue or frustration brought about by devotion to a cause, way of life, or relationship that failed to produce the expected reward. Stated another way: Whenever the expectation level is dramatically opposed to reality and the person persists in trying to reach that expectation, trouble is on the way* (Freudenberger, 1980).

> *Burnout is a syndrome of emotional exhaustion, depersonalization, and reduced personal accomplishment that can occur among individuals who do people work of some kind. It is a response to the chronic emotional strain of dealing extensively with other human beings particularly when they are troubled or having problems. Thus it can be considered one type of job stress. Although it has some of the deleterious effects as other stress responses, what is unique about burnout is that the stress arises from the social interaction between helper and recipient* (Maslach, 1982).

Burnout is defined as psychological withdrawal from work in response to excessive stress or dissatisfaction. Burnout is used to refer to the situation in which what was formerly a 'calling' becomes merely a job. One no longer lives to work but works only to live. In other words, the term refers to the loss of idealism, excitement, and a sense of mission in one's work (Cherniss, 1980).

Burnout is a progressive loss of idealism, energy, and purpose by people in the helping professions as a result of conditions of work (Edelwich & Brodsky, 1980).

Burnout is...*the result of the individual's inability to cope with job stress culminating in a deterioration of service provided to clients, and further manifesting itself in a variety of physical and psychological signs* (Mendaglio, 1982).

Two of these perspectives on burnout need further elaboration: Maslach's social psychological model and Cherniss' transactional model. Maslach's model is important because of its empirical base. It is based on her extensive survey of a variety of helping professionals. Her pioneering work culminated in an operational definition of burnout as embodied in the Human Services Inventory (Maslach & Jackson, 1981). This instrument depicts burnout as a syndrome of emotional exhaustion, depersonalization, and reduced personal accomplishment (see Figure 1). They view burnout as an occupational hazard of those who are engaged in *people work*. For Maslach, burnout is a unique form of job stress rooted in the relationship between provider (of a helping professional service) and a recipient (client, student, or patient). Despite her emphasis on the helping relationship as the source of burnout she seems to attribute equal importance to such issues as the structure of organizations.

FIGURE 1 MASLACH'S SOCIAL-PSYCHOLOGICAL MODEL OF BURNOUT

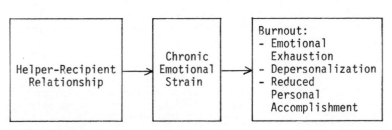

Cherniss' approach to burnout clearly is tied to the broader field of stress. His model is based on the transactional model of stress developed by Lazarus (1966) and Lazarus and Launier (1978). The work is notable in that burnout is seen as a subset of the broader notion of stress (see Figure 2). Lazarus' three-staged approach is evidence of the movement of the study of job-related stress reactions from an isolated phenomenon to a logical link with the broader area of psycho-social stress. In the first stage of Job Stress, an imbalance is experienced between the resources of the individual and the demands imposed by the job. Strain, the second stage, is seen as the individual's immediate reaction to the experience of stress. This is characterized by feelings of anxiety, fatigue, exhaustion. In the third stage, Defensive coping, the professional engages in a variety of self-defensive strategies such as detachment from clients, together with cynicism and rigidity.

FIGURE 2   CHERNISS - TRANSACTIONAL MODEL OF BURNOUT

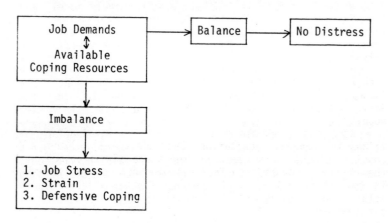

STRESS, JOB-STRESS AND BURNOUT

Two of the more popular approaches to stress are Selye's biochemical model (Selye, 1983) and Lazarus' transactional model as cited earlier.

FIGURE 3 SELYE'S BIOCHEMICAL MODEL

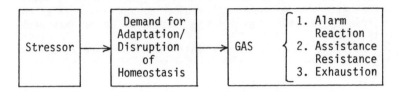

Biochemical Model of Stress

Based on his research on laboratory animals, Selye (1974) proposed a model of stress (see Figure 3) which is encompassed in the General Adaptation Syndrome (GAS). Prior to describing the three stages of GAS some basic terms have to be defined. *Stress* in Selye's view is any demand that is placed on an organism. A basic assumption is that stress can be both positive (*eustress*) or negative (*distress*) in nature. In either case, a stressor is something which disrupts the homeostasis of the organism. It must be emphasized the stress is not simply *nervous tension* (Selye 1974) but relates to the imbalance of the organism's homeostasis resulting from any demand for adaptation. In Selye's view, then, stress is an unavoidable, necessary part of life. In fact he claims that the absence of stress denotes death of the organism. Distress, on the other hand, is what needs to be reduced or managed. As can be seen, Selye's view of stress is rather different from the more popular usage.

For Selye, exposure to a stressor results in the triphasic General Adaptation Syndrome (GAS). The GAS consists of the alarm reaction, the stage of resistance, and the stage of exhaustion. The physiological changes embodied in both the alarm reaction and the stage of resistance relate to an increase in activity of the hypothalamus-pituitary-adreno-cortical axis. Persistent exposure to the stressor leads to exhaustion of the organism and may lead to death. However, it must be noted that not all stressors necessarily engage all three phases of the GAS, and, even in those instances where the third stage is experienced, exhaustion is not irreversible. Death results when adaptation energy of the organism is consumed. Selye claims that adaptation energy is finite and of two types: superficial and deep. Superficial adaptive energy is the type which can be readily restored through rest and relaxation. This daily renewal of superficial energy is achieved only through drawing upon the limited reserves of deep adaptation energy. One analogy to illustrate this notion of energy is as follows: consider a bank deposit being made at conception.

Genetic factors would be the *depositors*. As life progresses through the various developmental phases the individual makes withdrawals from the finite amount of adaptation energy. Life ends when all the adaptation energy has been withdrawn. Selye believes that all deaths are stress-related. In his view no one dies of old age per se.

Transactional Model of Stress

Lazarus believes that stress results from a complex interaction between the individual and the environment. The nature of stress is seen as the imbalance that occurs when the individual's resources available to deal with a demand are insufficient. If a demand (internal or external in origin) is placed on an individual and she/he perceives that means of meeting the demand are not readily available, stress occurs (see Figure 4). This is similar to Selye's usage of homeostasis, but it is a psychological equilibrium which is given greater emphasis by Lazarus.

The individual's interpretation of situations, events, and coping strategies, is central to Lazarus' theory. A central facet to the transactional model of stress is the individual's appraisal of situations/events (primary appraisals) and the resources available (secondary appraisals).

Lazarus places the individual's cognitive appraisal clearly at the vanguard of the stress experience. For Lazarus, stress is not to be found in an event nor in the individual but in the individual's *judgment that a transaction involves jeopardy (threat), harm-loss, or an opportunity to overcome hardship (challenge) by drawing upon more than routine resources* (Lazarus & Launier, 1978).

Lazarus discusses two general categories of coping strategies: *Active Problem Solving* and *Palliation*. In contrast to the task oriented category, *Palliation* refers to the application of strategies which essentially focus on the affective reactions associated with appraisals of stress. For example, strategies used to escape the situation (e.g., through drugs, alcohol) are palliative in nature.

The emerging conceptualization of burnout and job stress among helping professionals can readily be accommodated in Lazarus' theory of stress. As mentioned above, Cherniss has proposed a transactional model of burnout. Another example is the work of Pines et al.(1981), who clearly take an interactional view of burnout emphasizing that burnout is the result of bad situations and not *bad people*. Citing Lazarus' model, they developed a four-category approach to coping strategies which involve two dimensions: direct-indirect; active-inactive:

1. **Direct-active**: changing the source of stress, finding positive aspects in the situation.

2. **Direct-inactive**: ignoring the source of stress, avoiding the source of stress.

3. **Indirect-active**: talking about the stress, changing oneself to adapt to the source of stress, getting involved in other activities.

4. **Indirect-inactive**: drinking or using drugs, getting ill, collapsing.

FIGURE 4 LAZARUS - TRANSACTIONAL MODEL

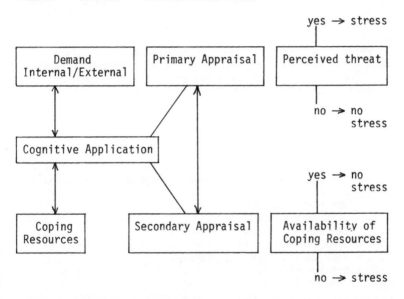

DEFINITION OF SALIENT CONCEPTS

Burnout

For the purposes of this chapter, burnout is seen as the end result of a helping professional's inability to cope with job demands. All professionals experience job stress but not all professionals are destined to experience burnout. Burnout and job stress are viewed in a transactional context: while the symptoms may be evident in the individual the source is accepted to rest in a complex interaction between the individual and the working situation.

Further, burnout is not viewed as transitory in nature, nor as an acute reaction (e.g., burnout is not simply having *a bad day at the office*), but as a chronic state manifesting itself in both negative psychological and physical reactions. Given that these negative reactions may have their origin in a variety of contexts (e.g., non-work stress in chronic medical conditions) it is essential to establish the source as being in the job, before organizational change is entertained and undertaken.

Stressors

While the delineation of organizational stressors is difficult, given the transactional context, researchers have attempted to identify stressors through self-reported questionnaires. The resulting data holds consistently across general response domains. It is these consistencies to which the topic of stressors is directed. An attempt is made to relate these stressors to the transactional context.
The literature reviewed has generated an extensive list of stressors in organizations:

- reality shock - discrepancies between the educational institution dogma and the real job setting,
- negative environments - punishment,
- negative reinforcement - employees directed to behave in specific ways to avoid punishment,
- rigidity in the environment - lack of opportunity to be creative,
- monetary issues,
- lack of autonomy,
- ambiguity and closure tension,
- negative public perceptions of the care-provider,
- lack of feedback and planning,
- heavy workload,
- role conflicts and ambiguity,
- too much paper work which prevent practitioners from exercising the service skills they were trained to deliver, and
- caseloads which reduce the time the practitioner can devote to doing an *adequate* job.

A variety of internal stressors have been identified as well:

- high order needs such as self esteem and self actualization unfulfilled,
- role confusion or diffusion,
- unrealistic or misguided goals, and

- practitioner's needs which are unmet through
organizational goals and responsibilities.

Consistent with Lazarus, the individual practitioner or
educator's secondary appraisal may lead the practitioner to
conclude he is *at risk*. It appears that the stressors
(internal and external) erode the self-concept and self-
esteem of the individual practitioner. In a general sense,
the stressors foster a sense of hopelessness, *inadequacy*,
and *ineffectiveness*. *This erosion of the practitioner's
self-perceptions of competence contributes to the phenomenon
termed burnout. Burnout has been referred to as the loss of
human caring. Possibly the loss of human caring is a
symptom of a more basic problem: the loss of self-efficacy
or perceived* lack of self-efficacy.

THE IMPACT OF STRESSORS

The Erosion of Self-efficacy in the Rehabilitation Practitioner

The variety of stressors identified suggests that stress is
a pervasive problem and should be observed in a contextual
focus of merging issues (Whitebrook, 1981). Added to this,
the responses to stress are multiple. Thus the likelihood
of predicting how an individual will respond to stress is
tenuous at best. The lack of predictability regarding an
individual's response to stress is analogous to the individual's response to the presentation of punishment which is
highly unpredictable (Martin & Pear, 1983). Through
extended exposure to punishment, the individual's responses
may be more generalized, exhausting and volatile leading to
the indirect-inactive expressions postulated by Pines. The
development of a taxonomy of stressors is likely, at best,
only to be able to identify the most obvious of stressors.
However, does the identification of stressors and the
removal of stressors as they are identified hold the solution to ameliorating burnout and preventing its occurrence
in the future?

If the researcher investigates the *social organization*
in concert with stressor identification, has he/she focused
more comprehensively on the phenomenon of burnout? It does
appear clear, at least, that stress is a response to loss of
self-esteem, loss of self-confidence, loss of self-worth and
erosion of self-efficacy. If the loss of self-efficacy is
the *focal* point of burnout, then a reasonable approach for
the researcher would be that of discovering how well the
organizational environment fosters the well-being of its
employees through the following questions:

1. Are there signs or signals in the environment which indicate that the practitioners are valuable and important to the organization?
2. Are there signs and signals in the environment which indicate to the practitioners that they are valuable and important to the organization?

In essence, does the situation *alarm* or does the situation promote performance through activities characterized by *delicious uncertainty*?

It appears that extremely positive responses to the above questions would indicate that the organization holds its individual practitioners in high regard and assumes, clearly, that they are vital to the organization. Additionally, the individual practitioner is not left in a vacuum of ambiguity - he or she knows that he/she is vital.

This section deals with a variety of stressors as identified at the beginning of this paper, together with examples. The discussion of each stressor will conclude with its impact on the self-efficacy of the practitioner.

DISCUSSION OF PROMINENT STRESSORS

Reality Shock

Reality shock programmes have been instituted to alleviate the stress of biculturalism reported by new graduate nurses (Hollefreund, 1981). The difficulty that many new graduate nurses face is that of interfacing their *schooled* values with the *work-setting* values. The reality shock programmes were designed to:

1) focus, with the new graduate nurses, on the nature of reality shock;
2) discuss the nurses' *current* efforts and actions as they relate to their professional nursing goals;
3) discuss feedback, feedback styles and how to give feedback;
4) discuss value systems (school versus work); and,
5) discuss in a culminating, all-day workshop, value differences, empathy training and conflict resolution.

The programme is multi-modal and, therefore, it is difficult to know which components were most valuable. It was, nevertheless, successful over a three year follow-up period which saw a reduction in attrition among new graduate nurses from an initial rate of over 30 per cent to less than 5 per cent (N=28).

What did the programme do? It appears that the programme was effective in several ways:

1. It enabled nurses to evaluate their feedback as compared with other comparable nurses - provided assurance to the nurse that her perceptions were not *unrealistic* and were shared by many peers;
2. It helped nurses focus on shared feelings and assisted in eliminating self-statements like *I'm all alone*.
3. Nurses were able to cope with the realities of conflict which had to be dealt with to a greater extent while on the job, as opposed to during the training each nurse received.

The programme then assisted nurses in generating positive *feelings* about their jobs, their careers, and themselves. Negative self-statements were tempered and nurses experienced high self-esteem, self-confidence, and self-efficacy. Nurses it appears were able to change the source of stress and find positive aspects in the situation (direct-active). It appeared that the Reality Shock Program increased communication about concerns, fostered a climate of caring, promoted a focus on real, presenting issues, and generated an atmosphere of mutual trust.

Negative Environments

Environments which have a preponderance of punishment or threat of punishment are unlikely to induce a satisfying self-concept within practitioners. These environments are like the adverse situations identified by Pines. Organizations which were set by senior management to coerce the people *below* to behave accordingly, are intimating that practitioners cannot think for themselves (much less be useful in establishing the climate and vision of the organization). This hardly seems a useful strategy if it is important to foster pride in the organization and the employees themselves. In this type of organization practitioners who choose to challenge the existing order and question the organization's motives are often exposed to extensive organizational censure and ridicule. Again, the growth of a *sense of self* and the sense of usefulness in one's role can be seriously deterred and even halted.

Related to this, when the practitioner's personal goals of rehabilitation and the organizational goals are in conflict, and there is no concomitant opportunity to *voice* the conflict, the stress levels increase. The individual practitioners, because they are unable to focus their aspirations or at least interface their aspirations through some form of synergistic dialogue, are faced with an inability to shape their own and their clients' futures. It is postulated that these environments may lead quickly to the indirect-inactive response to stress.

Rigidity

An overwhelming list of rules of order and conduct can be restrictive and stifling to the practitioner who is trained to provide optimal rehabilitative service (Mattaliano, 1982). Attempts *to right the ills* may often be inordinately delayed as the practitioner seeks *permission* to begin his/her treatment efforts. The practitioner may begin to feel the creativity generates *more work than it's worth* (Hyson, 1982). Realizing that the practitioner has been trained to deliver service, compounds the *uselessness* he or she comes to feel when faced with the multitude of tasks necessary to adhere to the protocol of the organization. Even the best prepared practitioner is unlikely to be able to endure the feeling of being ineffectual. The irony of rigidity is that the behaviours desired by most organizations are creativity and innovation and, yet many of these organizations have prevented their practitioners from being inventive. In fact these organizations may *teach* their employees to be active outside their vocation (indirect-active orientation). The labour of gaining approval and the risk of the project becoming something altogether unlike its original *vision* will effectively deter the practitioner from most forms of creative expression.

Negative Public Perceptions

Most people like to feel they are *valuable*, *doing a good job*, and *important to the community*. Attacking the practitioner's vocation prevents him/her from building a self-concept of worthiness which would include perception of *important to society* and *valuable community member*. Edelwich and Brodsky (1980) suggest that stress is generated through high public visibility which is paired with popular misunderstanding and suspicion. Failure on the part of the organization to make the public aware of their employees' value to society and the organization may seriously increase the stress under which the practitioner most operate (Huidekopfer, 1982). Compounding the problem for practitioners is the likelihood that they are public service employees, especially when there is a lack of public support for programmes (Gmelch & Swent, 1981). The media and cartoonists frequently, for example, make public service personnel the *brunt* of their criticisms - further lessening the practitioners' value.

Lack of Feedback

The parents or guardians of the clients entrusted to the practitioner also may experience a variety of stressors (Hoeppner, 1981). While practitioners, who are well-trained, may experience confusion, apprehensiveness and doubt, so may parents. In fact, the stress for parents may be more severe because they are *less-educated* about rehabilitation and education issues. Frequent feedback to parents (Hoeppner, 1981) is necessary where the *progress* of the learner is stressed. For example, a principal of a segregated school had teachers send home a monthly report on the child's *progress*. The cardinal rule enforced was that this letter, for each child, must stress the child's growth and that no mention of past progress, regression or untoward behavior exist.

Hoeppner (1981) further suggests that practitioners carefully ensure that the parents are *made to know* how important the job they are doing is to the education and rehabilitation of their child. Parents, like the practitioner, need to feel valued. Further emphasis must be given to ensuring that collaboration is mutually beneficial.

One of the ways that an individual practitioner generates a perception of *self* and *value of self* is through his or her efforts to facilitate client development. When development and growth of one's clients is interfaced with the goals of the organization, and is positively correlated, one might expect an increase in self-esteem. However, when client progress is less than optimal (not consistent with the goals established), the value one attributes to 'self' and his/her work is lessened (Freudenberger, 1977; Mattingly, 1977). When the goals of the organization cannot be achieved through the clients, the practitioner cannot experience success long enough, or for durations of any meaningful, significant consequence.

The practitioner who cannot facilitate the development of independent living skills in a mentally handicapped adult is not unlike the teacher who is frustrated because he/she is unable to develop problem-solving skills and responsibility which extends beyond the classroom. In each case the practitioner may *question* his or her capabilities as a service provider. Continued inability to gain optimal growth sequences in clients erodes the concept of *self*.

A second type of feedback comes from the significant managers in the organizational setting and is divided into two foci:

1) feedback which reflects to the practitioner his/her importance to the client; and,
2) feedback which reflects importance of the practitioner to the organization (Huidekopfer, 1982).

269

Feedback in the form of client progress (discussed previously) is not sufficient feedback even when client progress is optimal.

When feedback from managers is not present, the ambiguity of the *data* regarding a practitioner's performance can be confusing. The practitioner may be unable to interpret his or her confusion. The practitioner may be unable to interpret his or her *significance*. The practitioner is unable to pinpoint his/her *excellence* and may confirm, due to lack of data, that he/she is *valueless* (Dunham, 1980). The necessity to let employees know their value to the clients they serve and the value they have to the organization seems obvious if employees are to be fulfilled in their jobs. Without feedback employees may be seriously hampered in their attempt to appraise. Without primary appraisal can secondary appraisal be facilitated?

A third type of feedback, least well-addressed in the literature, is the self-generated feedback by the practitioner, *self-praise* and *self-deprecation*. Self-statements affect the way people behave. Some practitioners may have a learning history of self-deprecation; other practitioners may not attend to *all the data* regarding their performance and, in fact, focus only upon the *negative data*; and, a third practitioner may operate under an umbrella of irrational beliefs (e.g., I must never be wrong; making mistakes; show weakness; or have students fail in my classes). Individual practitioners need to learn to focus on all the evidence regarding their performance, develop *self-praise* and alter their beliefs to ensure that they are in line with more rational expectations. Researchers may do well to investigate the effects of Rational Emotive Therapy (RET) (Ellis, 1962), simulation training, imagery training, and cognitive behavioral strategies with practitioners in rehabilitative settings.

RET assumes that many emotional difficulties (it is implied here that stress encompasses such emotional reactions) are generated by irrational assumptions. The practitioner who believes it is of dire necessity to be loved by all his/her students for everything he/she does will undoubtedly find teaching stressful. Effective RET may generate a more reasonable set of assumptions for practitioners from which to operate. A specific RET strategy that is salient here is that of cognitive restructuring. The aim of this strategy is the replacement of faulty thinking with new, more rational view of reality.

Cognitive restructuring seems particularly useful when the imagery of the individual practitioner may foster stress. If the imagery is one of failure, inadequacy, and ineptness, the practitioner will likely be forced to endure large amounts of stress on a frequent basis. Strong imagery of success and an orientation to temporary setbacks (Orbick,

1980) as opposed to *failure* would go a long way to reducing stress. Practitioners and teachers, not unlike athletes or musicians, must see themselves as *winners*.

The application of cognitive restructuring with personnel in rehabilitative settings may have as much merit as the same strategies applied to one's clients.

Lack of Autonomy

Lack of control over one's environment may be very stressful. Seligman's research on both animal and human subjects suggests that repeated exposure to negative experiences beyond an individual's control leads to learned helplessness and depression (Seligman, 1979). In such cases, individuals attribute failure to themselves rather than to external factors. In a work setting this view suggests that bad situations may lead practitioners to incorrectly conclude that they are bad people.

The lack of opportunity to create one's dream, to realize one's vision, and to be *master of the path* (or at least some aspects of the road to rehabilitation) can be devastating. Consequently, the stealing away of autonomy from practitioners may have profound impact on the entire organization. Practitioners must see themselves as capable of influencing their work situation (Meadows, 1981).

Ambiguity/Role Tension, Role Conflict and Closure Tension

There are two types of role ambiguity:

1) that which occurs when the responsibilities assigned to the practitioner are unclear, opposing, or vague (Dunham, 1980; Iwanicki & Schwab, 1982; Bensky et al., 1980); and,
2) that which occurs when the practitioner is forced to select one treatment from a variety of treatment options.

The ambiguity of role definition prevents the practitioner from discerning the level of responsibility he/she can actualize. The tension (compounded daily) serves to exhaust the individual practitioner, as he/she always runs the risk of usurping administrative authority. The resultant feeling of *never can win* promotes a *keep your nose clean* approach to serving clients. System maintenance assumes greater priority than client growth and development.

Role conflict, the second type of ambiguity, very often occurs with newly graduated practitioners. The practitioner is placed in a position where he/she was trained to deal with Situation A in Manner Z, while his/her agency has chosen to deal with Situation A in Manner Y. The conflict arises from a lack of *match* between training institutions and the field to which the practitioner graduates. When a practitioner's skills (learned in *school*) do not match the field, the practitioner begins to question him or herself, the training programme and the validity of job-related behavioral repertoire (Miller & Roberts, 1979).

Closure tension occurs on a daily basis. The practitioner repetitively experiences the completion of intervention only to have to begin another intervention (Miller & Roberts, 1979). As a result the practitioner can *never-see-the-end*. The *graduation* of his/her clients may be viewed as too long in coming, or even impossible. This dilemma is compounded with current thoughts of *life-long follow-up*, as in some sheltered workshop or vocational agencies. When closure tension is viewed in this light, the merit of mental health days assumes a more prominent position in rehabilitative settings.

Paper Work and Time Management

All the complexities of time management and paper work can be found in rehabilitative settings. The inability to schedule the day (imposed by the organization or as a result of procrastination) (Mercer, 1981), prioritize objectives, sequence training in small units, cope effectively with interruptions, collaborate and co-operate in interdisciplinary service (Matteson & Ivancevich, 1982), and cope with the documentation and evaluation of the service itself add to the *stress* in rehabilitative environments (Anderson, 1981; Scully, 1981; Olson & Matuskey, 1982). An inability to *get-a-handle-on* the above noted activities brings further dismay to the practitioners. Role overload (Freudenberger, 1977) may seriously impair the motivations of the caring health services practitioner. The gradual erosion of competence and excellence immerses the practitioner in confusion rather than therapeutic client endeavors.

RECOMMENDATIONS

The rehabilitative settings impact heavily on the practitioner. Increasing mandates to ensure recognition of client's rights, government and organizational rules and regulations, paper work, and *ambiguities* have eroded the *self-confidence* of the practitioner. While many issues (i.e., clients' rights) should be conscientiously maintained, the organizational systems for rehabilitative personnel must ensure that the individual practitioner's position in the organization is well defined and expansive enough to allow for creative, innovative and independent functioning. It is likely that the practitioner needs a clear, well-defined mission from which to exercise autonomy and responsibility. This brief orientation would suggest that organizations should undertake the following activities to ensure the development of self-esteem, self-worth and self-confidence in its practitioners:

1. Institute *orientation* programmes which assist new practitioners in making the transition from *school* to *work*.
2. Establish a system for establishing organizational and individual performance standards in which individual practitioners may be fully involved, as opposed to *coercing from the top*.
3. An old adage, *catch people being good*, should be transposed from the classroom to the work setting, where the intent is to ensure that individual practitioners *are made aware* of their valuable contribution to the organization. *Catching all the mistakes* without a concomitant effort to reward the *excellence* in the people in the organization cannot foster self-worth and self-esteem.
4. Individual practitioners must be assured that they are a valuable resource and that they are integral to the growth and development of the organization.
5. Creative expression must be given license if the labours of habilitative efforts are to reach fruition. The creative excellence and innovative expressions of practitioners require a feeding ground - a nurturing environment. Rigidity only serves to stifle the energies.
6. Public education *by the organization* must be designed to foster an accurate perception of the day-to-day activities of the practitioner. Image-raising profiles must be developed through activities which clearly enhance the profession.
7. Feedback must be carefully arranged when the clients are likely to progress slowly.
8. Feedback must come from the organization's managers and be directed to the value of the practitioner, to his/her clients, and to the organization.
9. Practitioners need to learn to interpret the data regarding their client's success as *evidence* of their efforts. Careful attention to detail and the full spectrum of available data appears warranted.
10. Practitioners need to be assured by their organizations that they are valuable resources. But more than that, they need to know that they can be relied on to make autonomous decisions - that they are responsible

professionals and will be expected to foster positive growth within the organization.

11. The practitioner's role and responsibility must be clearly delineated to decrease the ambiguities.

12. Organizations and *schools for practitioners* must collaborate in the determination of training programmes which prepare practitioners for the field.

13. Mental health days, programme in-service and workshops must be ensured to allow the practitioner an opportunity to rejuvenate.

14. Time management strategies must be taught - probably most appropriately at the pre-service level. In-service activities could well augment the pre-service training.

CONCLUSIONS

This chapter has proposed that the critical variable in analyzing stress is neither the organizational structure, nor the individual employee but the transaction between the two. Hence, it is postulated that one may reduce stress among practitioners, through organizational change. Careful attention to organizational activities will clearly delineate the impact that organizational practices have upon self-esteem, self-worth and self-confidence. If individual practitioners are to become self-efficacious, the organizations must carefully design systems which foster a sense of *value* among their practitioners. The operationalization of the activities which facilitate autonomy and creativity have been delineated in *In Pursuit Of Excellence* (individual level) (Orbick, 1980), and *In Search Of Excellence* (Peters & Waterman, 1982). On an individual level, personal meaning, commitment and self-control, self-assessment, team harmony, and self-direction are articulated in *In Pursuit Of Excellence*. The organizations charged with the delivery of human services could enhance personal and organizational excellence if careful commitment to ensuring self-worth and confidence was ensured. Organizations must reinforce individual performance (practice of skills) while concomitantly providing the impetus for practitioners to pursue the *vision* and *mission* of the organization. A practitioners' skills will only influence the organization if the practitioner believes that he/she has the potential to have profound impact. The task of organizations is to promote and enhance the practitioners' *perceived* value to the clients and the organization.

REFERENCES

Anderson, D. A. (1981) 'Lifestyles/Personal Health: Care in Different Occupations,' *NASSP, 65,*(449), 36-39.

Bensky, J. M., Shaw, S. F., Gouse, A. S., Bates, H., Dixon, B., & Beane, W. E. (1980) 'Public Law 94-142 and Stress: A Problem for Educators,' *Exceptional Children, 47*(1), 24-29.

Cherniss, C. (1980) *Staff Burnout: Job Stress in the Human Services,* Beverly Hills, Sage.

Daley, M. R. (1979) 'Burnout: A Smoldering Problem in Protective Services,' *Social Work, 24,* 375-379.

Dunham, J. (1980) 'An Exploratory Comparative Study of Staff Stress in English and German Comprehensive Schools,' *Educational Review, 32*(1).

Edelwich, J. & Brodsky, A. (1980) *Burnout: Stages Disillusionment in the Helping Professions,* New York, Human Sciences Press.

Ellis, A. (1962) *Reason and Emotion in Psychotherapy,* Lyle Stuart, New York.

Freudenberger, H. J. (1974) 'Staff Burn-Out,' *Journal of Social Sciences, 30*(1), 159-165.

Freudenberger, H. J. (1977) 'Burnout: The Organizational Menace,' *Training and Development Journal, 31,* 26-27.

Freudenberger, H. J. (with Geraldine Richelsan) (1980) *Burn Out: How to Beat the High Cost of Success,* Bantam, New York.

Freudenberger, H. J. (1981) *Burn-out: The High Cost of High Achievement,* New York, Bantam.

Gmelch, W. H. & Swent, B. (1981) 'Stress and Principalship: Strategies for Self Improvement and Growth,' *NASSP, 65*(449), 16-19.

Hoeppner, G. (1981) 'Parents Burn-Out Too!,' *English Journal, 70*(4), 59.

Hollefreund, B. et al. (1981) 'Implementing a Reality Shock Program,' *The Journal of Nursing Administration, XI*(1), 16-20.

Huidekopfer, P. (1982) 'Hill Street Blues - About Us Too!' *English Journal, 71*(4), 34-35.

Hyson, M. C. (1982) 'Playing with kids All Day: Job Stress in Early Childhood Education,' *Young Children, 37*(2), 25-40.

Iwanicki, E. F. & Schwab, R. L. (1982) 'Perceived Role Conflict, Role Ambiguity, and Teacher Burnout,' *Educational Administration Quarterly, 23*(1), 60-74.

Lazarus, R. S. (1966) *Psychological Stress and the Coping Process,* New York, McGraw-Hill.

Lazarus, R. S. & Launier, R. (1978) 'Stress-Related Transactions Between Person and Environment,' in L. A. Pervin & M. Lewis (eds.), *Perspectives in Interactional Psychology,* New York, Plenum.

Maher, E. L. (1983) 'Burnout and Committment: A Theoretical Alternative,' *Personnel and Guidance Journal, 61,* 390-393.

Martin, G. & Pear, J. (1983) *Behavior Modification: What It Is and How To Do It,* New Jersey, Prentice Hall.

Maslach, C. (1976) 'Burned-Out,' *Human Behavior, 5,* 16-22.

Maslach, C. (1982) *Burnout: The Cost of Caring,* Englewood Cliffs, New Jersey, Prentice Hall.

Maslach, C. & Jackson, S. E. (1981) (MBI) *Maslach Burnout Inventory,* California, Consulting Lists Press.

Mattaliano, A. P. (1982) 'Time for Change: Theory X or Theory Y - What is Your Style,' *NASSP, 66*(456), 37-40.

Matteson, M. & Ivancevich, J. (1982) 'The How, What and Why of Stress Management Training,' *Personnel Journal, 61*(10), 768-775.

Mattingly, M. A. (1977) 'Sources of Stress and Burn-Out in Professional Child Care Work,' *Child Care Quarterly, 6,* 127-137.

Meadows, K. P. (1981) 'Burnout in Professionals Working with Deaf Children,' *American Annals of the Deaf, 126*(1), 13-22.

Mendaglio, S. (1982) 'Burnout: An Occupational Hazard of the Helping Professions,' *Journal of Practical Approaches to Developmental Handicap, 6*(2/3), 34-38.

Mercer, P. (1981) 'Stress and the Guidance Counsellor,' *School Guidance Worker, 37*(2), 13-17.

Miller, L. & Roberts, R. (1979) 'Unmet Counsellor Needs: From Ambiguity to the Zeigernik Effect,' *Journal of Applied Rehabilitation Counselling, 10*(2), 60-66.

Olson, J. & Matuskey, P. (1982) 'Courses of Burnout in SLD Teachers,' *Journal of Learning Disabilities, 15*(2), 97-99.

Orbick, T. (1980) *In Pursuit of Excellence,* Coaching Association of Canada.

Peters, T. J. & Waterman, R. H. (1982) *In Search of Excellence,* Warner Books, New York.

Pines, A., Aronson, E., & Kafry, D. (1981) *Burnout: From Tedium to Personal Growth,* New York, The Free Press.

Scully, R. (1981) 'Staff Support Groups: Helping Nurses to Help Themselves,' *The Journal of Nursing Administration, XI*(3), 48-53.

Seligman, M. E. (1979) *Helplessness: On Depression, Development and Death,* Freeman Press, San Francisco.

Selye, H. (1974) *Stress Without Distress,* New York, Signet.

Selye, H. (1983) 'The Stress Concept: Past, Present, and Future,' in C. Cooper (ed.), *Stress Research: Issues for the Eighties,* Toronto, Wiley & Sons.

Tiedman, D. V. (1979) 'Burnout and Copping Out of Counselling,' *Personnel and Guidance Journal, 57,* 328-330.

Time Magazine (1981) 'The Burning Out of Almost Everyone.' September.

Whitebrook, M. (1981) 'Who's Managing the Child Care
    Worker: A Look at Staff Burnout,' *Children Today*, 10,
    2-6.